CW00472718

Few diseases are [...] arthritis; few cause as much [...] of the one hundred and more arthritic diseases can be treated; some can also be cured. In simple language, the author explains the many complex issues of good arthritis care — accurate diagnosis, comprehensive treatment and follow-up.

While medication has an important part in the treatment, best results are obtained when the treatment involves not only the doctor, the physical and occupational therapist, but also exercise, diet, weight control, rest, and family support. The book explains the comprehensive nature of arthritis management.

The book dispels many misconceptions about how arthritis affects living a normal, healthy life. It gives specific exercises and practical tips to strengthen and keep active the different body-joints prone to arthritis.

The Author

Ada P. Kahn has a Master's degree in Public Health from Northwestern University Medical School, USA, and is a former member of the teaching faculty of the University of Health Sciences, Chicago Medical School and Columbia College, Chicago. She is a consultant to various pharmaceutical companies and medical associations. Her background includes affiliations with American Medical Association, the US Army Department of Medical History, and the US Department of Health and Human Services. She had worked with numerous health-related associations and organizations in educational capacities over the past 30 years.

She is a fellow of the American Medical Writers Association and has been published in international magazines including *Your Health and Fitness, Medical Record News* and *The Apothecary.* She has co-authored award winning Facts on File titles, *The Encyclopedia of Phobias, Fears and Anxieties, Midlife Health: A Woman's Practical Guide to Feeling Good,* and is the author of *Diabetes: Causes, Prevention and Treatment.*

Arthritis

Causes, Prevention and Treatment

Ada P Kahn
MPH

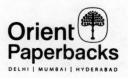

Orient
Paperbacks
DELHI | MUMBAI | HYDERABAD

www.orientpaperbacks.com

ISBN 13: 978-81-222-0134-5
ISBN 10: 81-222-0134-2

1st Published 1992
9th Printing 2007

Arthritis: Causes, Prevention & Treatment

Cover design by Vision Studio

Published by
Orient Paperbacks
(A division of Vision Books Pvt. Ltd.)
5A/8, Ansari Road, New Delhi-110 002

Printed in India at
Rashtra Rachna Printers, Delhi-110 092

Cover Printed at
Ravindra Printing Press, Delhi-110 006

Preface

Life starts with *movement* in the womb; and movement continues throughout life. Ageing shows its effect on movement in later life, and the aged person may even become crippled and bed-ridden under the effect of pain, deformity and immobility. Physiological ageing is an integral part of the growth process and both run parallel. Ageing joints show wear and tear and when symptoms of pain appear, *osteoarthritis* is said to have set in. Asymptomatic phase becomes symptomatic. Can ageing be arrested or stopped ? Possibly *no,* but it can be *delayed.*

The human locomotive system comprises of the axial skeleton (spine) and the limbs (upper and lower). Where two or more bones meet, a joint is formed (fibrous, cartilaginous or synovial). The articular surfaces are designed to provide movement (plane, hinge, pivot, condyloid, ellipsoid, saddle or ball-and-socket joints). Spine is a column of 33 bones and provides mobility and stability in humans unlike the animals where it acts as a suspension bridge. Each vertebral segment has a complex joint system with highly evolved weight bearing functions through intervertebral discs, facets and ligaments that any abnormality (even poor musculature and posture) results in *backache.* There is no individual who hasn't suffered from backache. If not today, it will come, tomorrow.

Pain, spasm, and loss of function are indications of joint malfunction. There is always a cause for pain. Whereas pain is a subjective phenomenon, spasm and loss of function are objective criteria; pain cannot be measured but spasm of muscles can be evaluated.

Arthritis is inflammation of the joints. Joint disease may start in the synovial membrane as an inflammatory process. It is mostly *rheumatoid arthritis* when it is of more than three months' duration and more than one joint is involved (more often polyarticular). An infective disease must be ruled out (tuberculosis is common in our country). Biopsy is essential and its importance should not be underestimated.

When the disease pathology starts in the articular cartilage it is called *osteoarthritis* and moves from early chondromalacia to destructive joint disease with severe deformities. Synovial involvement is secondary in this pattern of disease.

Diagnosis is the first step towards prevention of disease. An awareness of the abnormal functioning of the joint in the *asymptomatic* phase is necessary to prevent the development of osteoarthritis; rotational and angular deformities of the limbs predispose osteoarthritis. Excessive use and sports trauma lead to joint degeneration. Repeated bleeding in the joints is destructive. Overweight is certainly a contributory factor. Body is meant to be strong enough to withstand the day-to-day physical stress without developing any effective changes or signs of wear and tear. Light-weight, active life, regular fitness exercises to mobilise the joints through full range and tension-free lifestyle, are the basic essentials for healthy joints.

Rest to the painful joints, alternating with active, assisted and passive (controlled) mobilisation through a pain-free range, supplemented with range of motion and isometric exercises constitute the basic treatment which has both curative and preventive effects. Exercises should aim at developing *endurance* through regular isometric exercises, and *bulk* through resistance exercises. Heat (dry or wet) relieves pain (cold has a similar effect) and should be applied for about 10 minutes. Antiinflammatory creams and oil massage help in relieving the spasm. Such modalities can be carried out at home by the family members. Sophisticated equipment for physical therapy are available in physiotherapy centres. Splints to protect the joints can be made by the specialist.

Pain can be relieved through drugs : a) Steroids – the magic drugs which when given in a calculated dose for short periods give *hope* of the sufferer, but has the disadvantage of dependency and steroid complications due to prolonged use. Steroids can be injected into the joints also and their value is well established. b) Disease modifying drugs which are basically toxic in nature and require careful monitoring. They act slowly and take about three months to control the disease. c) Non-Steroid anti-inflammatory drugs which are much safer and can be used for longer periods. At present the emphasis is on single-dose drugs for better compliance. Pain relief is achieved through the anti-inflammatory action, and if still needed, analgesics can be supplemented for better comfort.

Combination of drugs should be carried out by experts. Joint disease with metabolic disorders may require special drugs. Drug therapy should not be used continuously for long periods for fear of gastric complications.

Rheumatic disease of childhood deserve a special note; as a variety of diseases have similar symptoms and pathology; and involvement of various connective tissues in the body at the same time. Certain other diseases have points of similarities to these disorders, and hence correct diagnosis is essential. Possibility of tuberculus arthritis must always be ruled out.

Surgery has a definite place in the management of arthritis. *Arthroscopy* is a diagnostic procedure and in addition to visual recording, synovial biopsy, removal of loose bodies and shredded pieces of meniscii that devides the cavity of a synovial joint can also be carried out. Arthroscopic surgery provides facilities for synovectomy and abrasive surgery in badly affected joints (knee). Joint replacement is at present a routine surgical procedure for hips, knees, shoulders, elbows, wrists and ankles.

Let us not forget the individual as a whole. An arthritic patient is *in pain all the time* and this affects his/her personality. They are often tense and stiff. They have disturbed sleep and are often irritable and not in physical or mental state to cope up with demands and stresses of life. Every family member has to *adjust* to the situation created by the presence of an arthritic member. Drugs alone cannot cure the sickness. Rehabilitation of an arthritic cripple is equally important; their mobility, participation and involvement in the family affairs must be preserved at all costs and efforts.

There is a genetic and hereditary factor involved in the development of arthritis, and an awareness of this possibility will help in prevention of arthritis in other family members by elimination of contributory factors, early diagnosis and treatment. Certain arthritic conditions (ankylosing spondylitis) still pose a challenge until a breakthrough comes in the near future.

Thus, while arthritis was once thought of as a disease you have to learn to live with – the present atmosphere is one of a groundswell of enthusiasm for the efficacy of current therapy and optimism for the future. In this book Ada P. Kahn captures this feeling of optimism and enthusiasm that now pervades the field of arthritis. In simple language the author deals with the many complex issues of arthritis so that virtually anyone can grasp the three essentials of good arthritis patient care. These are a) accurate diagnosis, b) comprehensive treatment and c) follow-up. Strict observance of these three essentials of arthritis care is the best way to assure the arthritis patient of optimal care. Books, such as this volume will continue to play an important role in helping arthritis patients understand that there is hope.

(Prof). Dr. J.S. Makhani
M.S. (McGill), FRCS (Canada), FACS
Formerly Head of Surgery
Maulana Azad Medical College, New Delhi.
Senior Consultant in Orthpaedic Surgery
Sir Ganga Ram Hospital
New Delhi.

Foreword

This book is intended to help readers better understand arthritis as a disease that takes many forms and can substantially alter one's feeling of well-being. The author has explained that while there are no cures for arthritis, there are many ways to help people who have arthritis to cope and improve their lives. Recognizing early signs and seeking appropriate treatment are important initial steps to feeling better.

In the past, the medical community did not consider arthritis as a significant illness. However, as the number of arthritis sufferers continues to increase, physicians and the public are taking notice of arthritis as a major illness. In fact, it is probably the most common complaint people make during office visits to their primary care physicians.

Today, people should not be complacent and just accept their arthritic pains. There are now specially trained physicians called rheumatologists who treat arthritis and its related conditions.

Until there is a cure for arthritic diseases, attention to self-help and lifestyle changes is essential. Although scientific advances have contributed to better understanding of the physiological processes at work to create arthritic pain and suffering, the medical community acknowledges the value of self-help and lifestyle changes to enable individuals to live more comfortably with arthritis.

This book offers an overview of types of arthritis and some suggestions for self-help, lifestyle changes, as well as help that can be obtained with the assistance of a physician. While self-help and lifestyle changes can contribute significantly to a patient's comfort, many individuals do require medical attention, and particularly a thorough diagnostic work-up, before embarking on a self-help and lifestyle change routine.

This book will help readers better understand their disease and the possibilities for relief. The important message throughout the book is that arthritis is not one, but many diseases; indeed there are over 100 different forms of arthritis. What works for one individual may not be effective for another individual. Even with excellent medical care, an individual may be asked to try several different medications and exercise routines before settling on one regimen that comfortably controls the individual's disease. Thus treatment of arthritis requires confidence is one's physician as well as *patience* with a prescribed regimen.

You'll read about the appropriate role of rest, exercise, diet, medications and surgery in arthritic diseases, as well as some suggestions for making each day easier. There is a special section for women and children with arthritis, as well as an excellent resource section which includes other books of related interest. A glossary defines many of the technical words used throughout the book.

Many people who have arthritic pains are frightened and need to talk with someone knowledgeable. After an initial consultation and thorough examination by a physician specially trained in rheumatology, to give the patient the best chance for improvement, I believe in a multi-disciplinary approach. The team approach utilizes a nurse coordinator, physical therapist, occupational therapist, social worker, and persons from other related disciplines as needed to help manage each case individually. The team can meet together and coordinate the patient's care, thereby giving the patient the best possible individualized care. In this way the patient can maximize his or her quality of life and learn as much as possible about the illness.

I caution people against believing in old *folklore* cures or new *miracle* cures that appear in television and in newspapers and magazines. Researchers are making progress every year in finding the various causes of arthritis. In the meantime, there is hope and arthritis sufferers will improve if they work closely with their physician and other members of the health care team.

Finally, I hope that readers of this book will gain a better understanding of their disease and make the best use of treatment by a physician as well as by self-help.

Dr. Robert A. Hozman, M.D.

Contents

If you have been told that you have arthritis, you probably have many questions about your disease, how it will affect your overall health, what your treatment will be and what you can do to help yourself to better health. While your physician and your health care team will be your best sources of information, this book will serve as an introductory handbook on the basics of the disease. If you have had arthritis for some time, you may regard this book as a refresher course concerning the disease.

This is not an encyclopedia about arthritis. Think of it as a handy outline that will help you learn more about your disease. Many other books on arthritis can be found on the health shelves in your local bookstores and libraries. Arthritis is a popular subject, and each book can contribute to your knowledge by discussing different aspects in varying degrees of detail. While you may know much of what is included in these books, if you learn only one new thing from each, your reading efforts will be rewarded.

The main theme that runs through this book is that there are ways you can help yourself to health while following your physician's treatment plan. What you do for yourself may be more important than—and is certainly as important as—taking your medication and appearing for physical therapy, if it has been prescribed for you.

Because controlling your arthritis is such a personal matter, participation on your part is essential to controlling your disease. You will want to learn all you can about arthritis. With a better understanding, you will be better able to follow your health care team's recommendations.

It is often hard to absorb and interpret everything that is explained to you when you are in a new health centre or when you are embarking on a new treatment programme. This book will also repeat some of the information you probably have been given by your doctor and other medical personnel and will help you follow your treatment routine appropriately. Additionally, this book will help you formulate any questions you might want to ask your doctor, nutritionist, or physical or occupational therapist during your next visit.

Much new information concerning arthritis has become available in recent years. If you read something here that differs from what you have heard from your health care team, discuss your questions with them. Ask how research developments may relate to your treatment plan. They will be able to advise you because they know you and your illness.

You will want to build a comfortable, efficient, working relationship with your health care team as you learn to control your arthritis. By following your health care team's recommendations, you *can* control your arthritis, as millions of others like you have done. You will work closely with your health care team to learn about medication, if it is prescribed for you, as well as about exercise, physical therapy, weight control, and following a well-balanced diet. These factors, together with a healthy mental attitude, can help you.

While researchers strive for improvements in treatment, you will want to keep yourself in the best possible physical condition so that you will be able to benefit from future innovations in treatment. You are the best one to control your daily diet, keep your weight at a healthy level for your age and body build, and incorporate appropriate exercise into your daily routine.

Arthritis takes many forms, but the type that affects most widely is osteoarthritis. Because it afflicts so many of us, this book will focus primarily on that type of the disease; rheumatoid arthritis, which also affects large numbers of people, is also discussed in some detail. The major types of arthritis will be explained briefly so that you will understand how your physician categorizes your disease and why.

How did you get arthritis? Why did you get it? What will your doctor do about it? What can you do about it? These and other questions will be addressed in an easy-to-understand style in the following chapters.

If someone you care about has arthritis, this book will provide information and useful hints on how you can help that person understand his or her disease and lead a healthier, more productive life. With your encouragement, your loved one will learn to follow professional health care advice and learn to live more comfortably with arthritis.

As you become better acquainted with arthritis you will want to increase your arthritis vocabulary. To help you incorporate the words relating to arthritis appropriately into your conversations with your doctor and health care team, a glossary has been included in this book. Also, a reading list and a list of sources available to those with arthritis are presented.

This book can help you in practical ways while you learn to follow your physician's instructions for taking care of yourself and your arthritis and helping yourself to health.

1

Arthritis: Your Personal Disease

Many people suffer the aches and pains of damaged or inflamed joints. Some are just uncomfortable, and some become crippled as a result of a disease that has been recognized since prehistoric times but understood in only the past few decades. The term *arthritis* covers a group of more than 100 diseases that involve inflammation of joints and discomfort in connective tissues throughout the body. In many parts of the world the disease is called *rheumatism*.

The *arth* part comes from the Greek word meaning joint, while *tis* means inflammation or infection. Thus the word arthritis means inflammation of the joint. The problem is that in many kinds of arthritis the joint is not inflamed. A better description might be *problem with the joint*.

You probably have known many people who have had arthritis and heard their stories of pain, of various attempts at treatment, and perhaps of some relief. Arthritis is a frequent conversational topic because it affects so many of us. It is estimated that about one out of every seven people in America have arthritis in some form.

People like to talk about arthritis because it is a very personal disease. It can be felt only by the person who has it, and often the symptoms can't be seen by others. Each person responds to treatment in different ways. Yet in few other diseases is there such a ready exchange of information by sufferers of the disease. Listening to others may be a good pastime but will not necessarily help you control your disease. As you learn more about arthritis you will understand why following your health care team's recommendations is important to obtaining relief and helping yourself to health. Your therapy programme will be individualized for you. The treatment that worked for your neighbour may not work for you, and vice versa.

The best counsel one arthritis victim can give another is to obtain competent medical advice. Seek treatment when symptoms are detected. Treatment is effective when begun before symptoms become associated with destruction of the joints.

In the following chapters you will learn more about how your doctor and health care team will diagnose your disease, plan a treatment programme for you, and work with you in following through with a combination of therapies to help you continue to lead a healthy, productive life.

Getting Acquainted with Arthritis

Aches and pains are called different things by different people, but when doctors say *arthritis,* they are referring to painful inflammation in a joint. In some forms of arthritis the inflammation brings with it swelling, pain and redness. The damage occurring in bones and tissues of the joints makes them stiff and often makes movement difficult.

Arthritis may be a chronic disease, as opposed to an acute disease, which is serious for a while, is treatable, and goes away with treatment. Some forms of arthritis do not go away but can be controlled with treatment. Treatment can help you lead a normal life and continue your daily activities in a productive way. The treatment for arthritis must continue. In many cases remission occurs. That means the symptoms disappear for a while but may reappear after some time. Treatment must be continued to prevent recurrence or to lengthen the amount of time before symptoms flare up again.

Most Common Forms

The most common forms of arthritis are osteoarthritis and rheumatoid arthritis. In the US over 16 million people have osteoarthritis, and about 6 million have rheumatoid arthritis. Osteoarthritis is sometimes known as the *wear-and-tear disease* or *old age arthritis*. It is solely a disease of the joints that occurs with increasing frequency with age, though it does affect people as early as age 35. It begins gradually and may remain mild for some time. There is usually little inflammation with this type of arthritis, and it does not cause general illness or affect parts of the body other than the joints. Disability often develops gradually.

Rheumatoid arthritis is inflammatory and attacks more than the joints. It may cause disease in the lungs, skin, blood vessels, eyes, spleen, and heart. This is a type of arthritis that can cripple and even kill. It is a chronic disease, but in some cases acute spells occur when inflammation flares up unpredictably. About three times more women have this type than men. In children it may destroy joints and can affect the growth pattern.

Three other types of arthritis are much less common. Ankylosing spondylitis is a chronic inflammatory condition most common in men, which affects the spine and usually begins in the teens or early twenties. Systemic lupus erythematosus (known as SLE or lupus) is an acute systemic disease related to rheumatoid arthritis. It causes inflammation and damage to joint and organs throughout the body. Sometimes the kidneys, heart, lungs, brain, and blood vessels are affected by inflammation. A common feature of the disease is a skin rash on the face. Ten times more women have SLE than men. Gout, or gouty arthritis, attacks and inflames any of the joints, one at a time. The most common site is the big toe. More men have it than women. For more details on arthritis see Chapter 2.

Early Warnings of Arthritis

Knowing how the types of arthritis differ will help you understand your disease and will help you work more effectively with your health care team. Aches and pains in and around joints can mean many different things——not necessarily arthritis. That is why it is important to be diagnosed as soon as possible after signs or symptoms appear. What are the signals of arthritis ? According to the US National Arthritis Foundation, there are four major warning signs :

1. Persistent pain and stiffness on arising
2. Pain, tenderness, or swelling in one or more joints
3. Recurrence of these symptoms, especially when they involve more than one joint
4. Recurrent or persistent pain and stiffness in the neck, lower back, knees and other joints

Looking at this list of warning signs, some people may think they have arthritis when they do not. For example, stiffness in the neck muscles is not necessarily arthritis but may actually be a result of sleeping in an awkward position. Soreness in muscles probably doesn't indicate arthritis when you have spent the previous day raking leaves. Many such discomforts disappear by themselves. When pain does not disappear, however, or when it recurs frequently, arthritis may be suspected. The only way to be sure is to have a complete physical examination and some specific tests' which your physician will recommend.

Diagnosis and Treatment

The first step involves a complete health history and examination. Diagnosis of arthritis is not easy because many of the signs and symptoms are similar in several arthritic diseases. Your physician may employ blood, urine, and joint fluid tests along with X-rays and other examinations. These tests will help your physician make a diagnosis.

The causes of your arthritis may be known or unknown. Although research has made great advances in the past few decades, much about the causes of arthritis remains a mystery. Yet much can be done to control arthritis. Physicians know that certain medications, including aspirin, help reduce inflammation and thus provide relief from pain. Other medications may actually inhibit the progress of rheumatoid arthritis. Physical therapy and exercise are often recommended to keep joints and muscles mobile and strong. Weight loss is frequently recommended when arthritis affects weight-bearing joints. In some cases surgery may provide relief and enables people to lead healthier, productive lives. Proper diet, relaxation, and a good mental attitude are also components of all treatment plans.

Based on the results of your examinations and tests, your diagnosis will include your individualized treatment plan. You will be advised to work closely with your physician to learn how to combine medication, exercise, diet and relaxation in your lifestyle so that you can help yourself towards health.

Your Lifestyle and Arthritis

In the early stages of treatment you may be advised to make slight changes in your lifestyle to accommodate some new routines of daily living. These may mean additional exercise, physical therapy, a diet planned to help you lose weight, and medications. You may try one medication and then be advised to change to another one. Such efforts will be aimed at developing the treatment plan that works best for you. Your doctor, physical therapist, nutritionist, and any other members of your health care team will make valuable contributions to your care.

At this time patience, understanding, and optimism will also be necessary components of your plan. Your health care team will explain that it takes time for treatments to work. Sometimes results are not noticeable right away.

Your health care team will also discuss with you the possible role of family and friends. You will find the love and consideration of those who care about you, helpful as you follow your treatment plan for arthritis. Health care professionals know the importance of having others around to carry out activities that require stronger hands and faster legs. You can look at ways to retain your independence while working as a team with loved ones to help you to better health.

Each person with arthritis has special concerns. Men and women worry about being able to keep their jobs and provide incomes for their families. Parents are concerned about being able to care for their children adequately: If disabling features of the disease appear, concerns deepen, and at such times health care professionals can provide valuable suggestions for living a normal life with arthritis. Suggestions may include utilizing many available helpful devices, aids and appliances and the services of community agencies. For details see Chapters 8 & 12.

Children with arthritis are concerned about being different as well as about being ill. All children want to enjoy the normal childhood pleasures. Arthritic children need the support of the professional health care team as well as those who love them to enable them to develop as normally as possible.

In later chapters you will learn more about special concerns regarding arthritis.

Save Money: Treat Arthritis Early

If you think you have arthritis or that someone about whom you care has arthritis, it is important for a diagnosis to be made early. If a diagnosis has been made, it is important to follow the advice given by the health care team. You can save money and spare yourself pain and anguish by following recommendations right away and helping yourself in the early stages of the disease.

Arthritis can be an expensive disease, but it need not be. It is expensive because it affects so many people in so many ways. Most people can live comfortably and continue to provide for themselves and their families. Others must cut down on the amount of work they do, change jobs, or stop working altogether. According to the US Arthritis Foundation, the annual cost to the national economy due to arthritis, in lost wages and medical bills, runs into billions of dollars. The cost in human suffering, pain, and disability can not be measured.

Following your doctor's recommendations can also help you save money on medication and therapies. Arthritis sufferers spend millions of dollars each year on quack remedies, only to be disappointed with the results. The medical profession won't hold any secrets from you when a real cure for arthritis is found. If the quack remedies were really safe and effective, the doctors you know would be recommending them to you. The US Arthritis Foundation maintains a misinformation file containing thousands of quack remedies for arthritis. Many won't hurt you, but they probably won't help either.

One of the dangers of using quack remedies for arthritis without consulting your physician is that you might be givng up a more effective treatment by following something that hasn't been proven to help in cases such as your own. In the long run you can do irreparable harm to yourself. Some advertised arthritis clinics may use remedies that have effects throughout the body that may be life threatening to certain individuals. When you read about a new breakthrough treatment for arthritis, discuss it with your physician. Your physician will know how it might influence *your* arthritis.

Arthritis, the Future, and You

You can be hopeful that therapies for treating arthritis will continue to improve. International research efforts indicate that an optimistic view of the future is a realistic one. Much has been learned about the causes and treatment of the disease in the last 30 years. Advanced research techniques are hastening development of treatments that will help arthritic patients.

While there is still no *cure* for many forms of arthritis, much research is being aimed at looking for potent therapies that will put the disease in remission with a minimum of side effects. Additionally, there are now ways to identify certain people who have genetic predisposition to arthritis. In other efforts scientists are looking at a particular type of white blood cell as a clue to a possible cause for arthritis. Analysis of certain viruslike organisms that may contribute to arthritis is being pursued by many scientists.

In Chapter 11 you will learn more about the advances in arthritis research and the new therapies that can provide your physician with more choices regarding your treatment.

Better understanding of the causes of arthritis and the treatment, combined with what you can do for yourself, can help you lead a more normal, productive life despite arthritis.

2

What is Arthritis?

Your body's joints are not like the joints of a robot. They can't be oiled when they feel stiff. Yet the joints in your body are mechanical parts, and when they no longer move easily and smoothly, they do not work effectively and comfortably. What causes the pain? What causes the stiffness? What can you do about it?

The first thing to get out of the way is the myth that there is such thing as a single disease called arthritis. The truth is that the word arthritis is about as useful and specific as the word infection; and just as there are over hundred different types of infection so there are over a hundered different types of arthritis.

Because arthritis takes many forms, some with devastating effects on your future health, careful diagnosis as soon as symptoms are noticed, is important. Early detection and prompt treatment can help relieve pain and prevent later complications. Arthritis affects individuals in different ways. Treatments that work for one person with one type of arthritis do not always work for another person with another type. Self-diagnosis and self-treatment, based on the experiences of others, can have potentially harmful effects in that it causes the self-medicator to postpone more appropriate, individualized treatment.

If you have symptoms of arthritis, you can help yourself by seeking prompt medical attention and diagnosis. If someone you love thinks he or she has arthritis, encourage the person to have a professional diagnosis and begin treatment.

Knowing more about the various types of arthritis will help you understand the disease and how you can help yourself while following the treatment plan outlined by your physician.

OSTEOARTHRITIS: The Wear-And-Tear Disease

Osteoarthritis affects more people than any other type. Physicians may refer to it as *degenerative joint disease*. Patients usually know this disease best as *old age arthritis*.

Why does osteoarthritis occur ? In a normal joint a smooth, elastic material called *cartilage* covers the ends of your bones where they meet. Cartilage enables the bones to glide smoothly across each other and gives joints their flexibility.When the cartilage wears away, it becomes painful to move the joint. The ends of the bones may develop spurs, or outgrowths, and ligaments and membranes around the bones may thicken. As a result the shape and structure of the joint may change. In reaction to the pain, muscles near the joint may become tense and contract. As muscles weaken, use of the joint may become more restricted. While each case of osteoarthritis is different, your understanding should begin with the anatomy of bones and joints.

While osteoarthritis can occur in any joint, the joints most commonly affected are the weight-bearing ones: knees, hips, and lumbar spine. It often affects the joints of the fingers, the base of the thumb, and the big toe.

Physicians categorize cases of osteoarthritis as primary and secondary. The primary form seems to begin by itself, with no specific cause, while the secondary type may have many causes but often results from too much stress and strain on a joint. Primary osteoarthritis occurs mosly in women and may have a hereditary component because it seems to appear more in some families than in others. It sometimes begins fairly early in life,

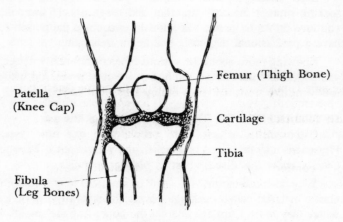

Patella (Knee Cap)

Femur (Thigh Bone)

Cartilage

Tibia

Fibula (Leg Bones)

The Knee Joint

even during the late thirties and early forties. Osteoarthritis seems to be quite generalized and affects small joints such as the fingers and toes.

What Causes Osteoarthritis?

Arthritis researchers don't have clear explanations of the causes of osteoarthritis. They believe multiple causes influence the development of the disease. The normal ageing process is one. Hidden birth defects may be another. Heredity may also be a factor, especially in the development of primary osteoarthritis.

Research efforts are under way to learn more about causes of arthritis, particularly osteoarthritis, as it affects many people. You will read more about research efforts in Chapter 11.

Do occupation and lifestyle relate to osteoarthritis? Researchers say that when joints are repeatedly stressed in the same way, osteoarthritis is more likely to develop. For example, a dock worker who bends and lifts all day is more likely to get osteoarthritis in his knees than an accountant who sits at a desk. A football player is more likely to develop osteoarthritis in his knees than a chess player.

How does Osteoarthritis Feel?

If you have osteoarthritis, your answer may be a woeful sigh. Osteoarthritis can hurt. The major symptom is pain, in and around joints. In different individuals the type of pain varies. It may be a constant aching, a feeling of soreness, or a more severe pain when you move your joints. The pain occurs because pressure is placed on the nerve endings due to the deterioration of the smooth cartilage between the bones. Tense muscles may also contribute to your discomfort. Sometimes the pain may radiate to other muscles that seem unrelated to your sore joint.

Another symptom is a reduced capacity for moving sore joints comfortably. This problem is compounded when muscles around the joint are weak.

You may be like many who have osteoarthritis, in that others can't tell that you have it. Only your inability to move some of your joints smoothly may be noticeable. However, in more severe cases, joints have a knobby look because changes have occurred in the bones with the disintegration of the cartilage covering them.

How is Osteoarthritis Diagnosed?

Sometimes osteoarthritis is detected on X-rays taken for other purposes. In this case, people may not feel any aches or pains but may be told by their physician that they have osteoarthritis. Often if a person complains of pains in joints, the physician will order X-rays because damage to a joint may be seen that way. However, X-rays are only part of the procedure your physician will follow to diagnose osteoarthritis. The history of your symptoms and the findings of the complete physicial examination also will be valuable factors in the diagnosis. Your explanation of how you feel will be very important. For example, persons with osteoarthritis usually do not have a feeling of being ill, do not experienece severe weight loss, and do not have a poor appetite or fever. Also, the pain in the involved joint is usually maximal with activity (walking, etc.) and decreased by rest in patients with osteoarthritis.

How is Osteoarthritis Treated?

There is no cure for osteoarthritis. The goal of therapy is to control the disease and possibly slow its progress by keeping the affected joints mobile, preventing further disability, and relieving pain. In some cases drugs, special exercises, rest, and heat are effective.

If you have osteoarthritis, depending on your symptoms, your physician may suggest avoiding physical activities that strain your sore joints. You may be advised to avoid occupational and recreational use of the affected joints. If weight-bearing joints are involved, you may be told to avoid weight-bearing activities such as climbing stairs or prolonged standing.

In other cases, orthopaedic surgery and rehabilitation therapy are helpful. How surgery helps some people with osteoarthritis will be explained in Chapter 5.

Sometimes drugs are injected directly into the joint affected by osteoarthritis. Some people obtain temporary relief from pain and disability in this way. Use of drug therapy in osteoarthritis will be explained in the next chapter.

If you are overweight, your physician will probably suggest a weight-reducing diet. Reducing weight will help reduce the strain on your joints, particularly if your osteoarthritis is in the hips or knees. In Chapter 7 you will learn more about how to lose weight to help control your osteoarthritis.

In some cases, physicians recommend traction, which involves stretching the upper part of the spine in the area of the neck, as a treatment for spinal osteoarthritis. In other cases physicians recommend using a neck collar or a heavy towel wrapped around the neck to support the weight of the head, thereby allowing the painful muscles to relax. These techniques provide relief but do not influence the progress of the disease.

What is the Outlook?

Prompt, appropriate treatment usually greatly relieves symptoms and improves function. Activity need not be permanently limited if control of the disease is maintained through the many techniques now available to your physician.

Researchers are constantly striving for additional means of controlling the disease and, ultimately, a cure.

RHEUMATOID ARTHRITIS: The Inflammatory Disease

Rheumatoid arthritis usually begins slowly but sometimes comes on suddenly. Symptoms may appear, go away, and return again. While it is a systemic disease of inflammation, the most noticeable symptoms are vaguely or acutely sore joints of the hands and feet. The inflammation also affects the connective tissues throughtout the body, which may contribute to a *sick all over* feeling.

Rheumatoid arthritis begins with inflammation in the synovial membrane, a thin tissue that lines the capsule surrounding the joint. Inflammation of the synovial membrane may spread to other parts of the joint. Inflamed tissue may grow into the cartilage surrounding the bone ends, causing it to deteriorate. When the cartilage disintegrates, scar tissue forms between the bone ends. Sometimes the scar tissue solidifies into bones, fusing the joint, making it rigid and difficult to move.

How Does Rheumatoid Arthritis Feel?

Different people have different symptoms, but characteristically pain and stiffness occur in the morning and subside during the day. If you have this disease, getting up in the morning may be the hardest part of the day for you. While a few minutes of stiffness in the morning may be normal, people with inflammation due to rheumatoid arthritis are frequently stiff for one or two hours.

Usually more than one joint is affected by rheumatoid arthritis. As the joints stiffen, swelling and tenderness become more appartent. Full motion becomes painful and difficult. When rheumatoid arthritis affects the hands, the fingers may become deformed and everyday tasks become difficult to perform. The pain may become more severe with strenuous activity.

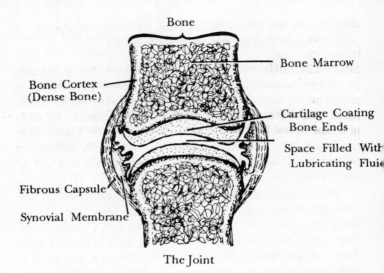

Bone

Bone Marrow

Bone Cortex
(Dense Bone)

Cartilage Coating
Bone Ends

Space Filled With
Lubricating Fluid

Fibrous Capsule

Synovial Membrane

The Joint

Because rheumatoid arthritis often affects connective tissues throughout the body, there maybe fever, poor appetite, weight loss, and anemia. The spleen and lymph glands may become enlarged.

Early diagnosis and treatment can reduce the possibilities of dangerous and crippling effects.

What Causes Rheumatoid Arthritis?

While rheumatoid arthritis may begin at any age, it most commonly affects people between the ages of 20 and 40. The cause of rheumatoid arthritis is not known. Some researchers say it is caused by infection. Heredity is definitely a factor. There is some agreement among researchers that the body's immune system is somehow involved in the development of rheumatoid arthritis.

Researchers believe that there is a foreign substance that may contribute to the development of rheumatoid arthritis, but they haven't isolated it yet. Inflammation induced by this foreign substance is thought to be responsible for the joint pain, swelling, and destruction so commonly seen in patients with this disease.

How is Rheumatoid Arthritis Diagnosed?

If this disease is suspected, your physician will find several laboratory tests helpful in addition to a complete physical examination, a health history, and X-rays. A test called the *erythrocyte sedimentation rate (ESR)* will indicate the presence of any inflammation in your body. You need only have a small blood sample drawn; then the depth that the red blood cells sink in a tube in one hour is recorded. Another test done with your blood sample helps determine the presence of rheumatoid factor, an abnormal antibody present in most people who have rheumatoid arthritis. In normal conditions the presence of abnormal antibody is nil. While rheumatoid factor may be present in people without rheumatoid arthritis, if symptoms of arthritis are present, the additional information regarding rheumatoid factor will be a useful diagnostic tool for your physician. For details see Chapter 3.

How is Rheumatoid Arthritis Treated?

Most physicians take a conservative approach to treating rheumatoid arthritis because they believe such management offers the best long-term results. The goals of therapy are reduction of inflammation and pain, preservation of function, and prevention of deformity.

Therapeutic programmes for people with rheumatoid arthritis are individually designed, depending on the extent of the disease and the organs involved. If you have rheumatoid arthritis, your treatment may include a mix of exercise and rest; use of heat, cold, or both; anti-inflammatory and remission-inducing drugs; possibly surgical repair; and in some cases use of special braces or other supports. You will learn more about specific therapies, such as the use of drugs, in Chapter 4. Treating your arthritis with lifestyle changes will be described in Chapters 8, 9 and 10.

Treatment for rheumatoid arthritis is usually developed by a team of health care professionals who work together to create the best possible programme for your care. Physical therapists, occupational therapists, rehabilitation specialists, and social workers will co-operate with your physician in planning and carrying out your treatment programme. Family members may become involved because love and emotional support can help relieve stress; and practical support, such as in doing household chores, maybe required to maintain the family's normal routine.

What is the Outlook ?

While the course of rheumatoid arthritis is unpredictable, excellent therapy is now available to reduce the inflammation and to reduce a drug-induced remission of disease activity. Sometimes permanent remission or disappearance of symptom, occurs. Thus, even if rheumatoid arthritis does not go into a natural remission, drugs are available to induce a remission.

OTHER FORMS OF ARTHRITIS

Ankylosing Spondylitis

In this type of arthritis the small joints of the spine and the sacroiliac joints are affected first. Pain in the lower back and legs is often one of the first symptoms. The hips and shoulders may become involved. The spine may become progressively stiffer. If untreated, the spine may develop such a curvature that the sufferer must stand in a stooped position. Delayed or inappropriate treatment can make this one of the most crippling forms of arthritis.

This disease differs from osteoarthritis of the spine in several ways. First, it often affects young adults between the ages of 20 and 30. It affects more men than women. This is an inflammatory disease, whereas osteoarthritis is a non-inflammatory disease. In ankylosing spondylitis complications can involve the eyes, heart, and, in rare cases, the lungs. About one-quarter of the people with this disease have eye complications. These can be controlled if detected and treated early.

If the disease progresses very far up the spine, the ribs can also became involved at the point where they join the spine, and this reduces the sufferer's ability to breathe because of the constriction of the lungs. Chest infection is then an ever present possibility. The jaws may be affected causing difficulty in eating and speaking.

Early diagnosis and treatment of ankylosing spondylitis often permits control of the disease, with avoidance of a great deal of discomfort and the possibility of deformity. The disease usually runs its course in several years. Although some stiffness may remain after a few years, the disease does not become progressively worse, as do certain arthritic conditions.

While the cause of ankylosing spondylitis is unknown, heredity is a major factor. About 90 per cent of all people with this disease have a genetic marker known as HLA B27. While many people have this genetic marker, however, not all of them will develop this disease. For details see Chapter 11.

Osteoarthritis and Spondylosis or Prolapsed (slipped) Disc

Whereas osteoarthritis is a degenerative joint disease which develops most commonly in the larger weight-bearing joints— chiefly the hips, knees, or spine of older people, prolapsed disc and spondylosis are also sometimes confused with arthitic diseases because these conditions are also the result of degenerated vertebrae. The only relation between osteoarthritis and spondylosis or prolasped (slipped) disc is the degenerative factor. Spondylosis or prolapsed disc are not arthritic diseases. These conditions can occur even due to injury or over straining.

Gout

Gout develops only after years of elevation of serum uric acid. The high uric acid level (The normal range of uric acid in blood serum is 3.0 to 6.0 mg per 100 ml) sometimes results from a hereditary defects in the body chemistry or after use of certain types of medications. Only about one out of 10 people who have an elevation of serum uric acid develop needle-like crystals in their joints, which lead to the severe inflammation, swelling, and tenderness, characteristic of gout. Although gout can affect almost any part of the body, the large joint of the big toe is usually attacked first.

Gout can be controlled very effectively. Treatment calls for medications directed at reducing the level of uric acid in the

Corelations of Arthritis

Signs/Symptoms	Rheumatoid Arthritis	Osteoarthritis	Arthritis Due to Specific Infection	Gout
Family History	Often.	Often.	No.	Often.
Sex	Most common in women.	Either Sex.	Either sex.	Most common in men.
Age at Onset	Any age, but usually 20-40.	Usually over 40.	Any age	Usually Over 35
Onset	Insidious (subacute), usual, acute, atypical.	Insidious (slow)	Acute infection: sudden, chronic infection slow.	Sudden (improvement of symptoms also sudden).
Fever	Occasionally.	No.	Yes (especially acute).	Occasionally during acute episodes.
Chills	Only in children.	No.	Yes	No.
Joints Involved	Involvement of small joints of hands and feet, especially proximal finger joints.	Usually the large weight-bearing joint; also end joints of fingers.	Most often the knee or shoulder.	Joint at base of great toe (bunion joint).
Muscle Atrophy	Yes.	No.	Yes (local).	No.
Deformities	Yes.	Yes (local).	Yes (late).	Yes (late).
Skin Changes	Thin and shiny over joints	No.	No.	Local scaling and itching with recovery from acute attack.

system, thereby preventing subsequent attacks of gout. For details on drugs used, see Chapter 4. While dietary changes were once a mainstay of gout treatment, the effectiveness of the medications in lowering serum uric acid now makes special diets unnecessary.

Systemic Lupus Erythematosus (SLE)

This disease may damage many tissues throughout the body, such as the joints, internal organs, and skin. It occurs more often in women than in men, and while it occurs most often between the ages of 20 and 30 it can occur at any age. SLE is like rheumatoid arthritis in that it may show periods of improvement as well as those in which it flares up. Symptoms—including joint pain, fatigue, weakness, kidney problems, loss of weight, fever, and skin rash—appear in different combinations. In most cases the disease can be controlled, but not cured. It is important for people with SLE to remain under the close supervision of a physician to help avoid serious complications. SLE seems to affect people in many different ways, and many treatments are used, depending on the individual. Generally, rest and medication are advised, together with drugs to reduce inflammation.

Arthritis as a Result of Infection

Acute or chronic arthritis can occur when bacteria get into the joints. This has been known to occur along with tuberculosis, meningitis, and gonorrhea. Fortunately, this type of arthritis can be halted after laboratory tests identify the bacteria and appropriate antibiotic treatment is given.

Rheumatic Fever

This disease is considered a form of arthritis because it inflames joints as well as damages the heart. Caused by a streptococcus infection, it can be treated with antibiotics and aspirin and usually clears up completely. The arthritis is painful but does not cripple.

Psoriatic Arthritis

Some individuals who have psoriasis — i.e. a chronic skin disease involving scaly patches on the body, especially the elbows, knees, scalp and neck— also have a variety of rheumatic diseases, and thus their arthritis sometimes is referred to as psoriatic arthritis. Symptoms are mild and individuals usually do not require very much treatment. Major symptoms of psoriatic arthritis are sorenes of fingers or other joints, and backache. In some cases, the joints at the ends of the fingers are swollen, and the fingernails become pitted and thickened.

While the disease affects men as well as women, and people of all ages, it is more common in women and usually occurs between the ages of 20 and 30.

Another type of psoriatric arthritis is known as spondylitis, and occurs primarily in the spine. This disease is very closely related to ankylosing spondylitis.

CONDITIONS WHICH MAY
SEEM LIKE ARTHRITIS BUT ARE NOT

Many discomforts of joints seem to resemble arthritic conditions because of their pain and discomfort. Indeed, some of the treatments used for them are similar to arthritis treatments. However, they are not considered arthritis.

Among this category of disorders are fibrositis and fibromyalgia, bursitis, tennis/golfer's elbow, frozen shoulder, housemaid's knee, baker's cyst, and Achilles' tendinitis.

Fibrositis and Fibromyalgia

The terms *fibrositis* and *fibromyalgia* refer to painful conditions that are technically not arthritis; they are conditions of the soft tissue, sometimes refered to as non-articular–soft-tissue rheumatism because joints usually are not affected. Individuals who have these syndromes experience stiffness, unexplained pain around their joints, a generalized feeling of aching, easy fatiguability, and sleep disturbances. While the patient may describe joint pain, physcians usually do not see swelling of joints during examinations. Some patients describe numbness, tingling and poor circulation. A physician may diagnose fibrositis by locating the existence of *tender points* throughout the body during a physical examination.

Many more women—a nine to one ratio—than men have fibrositis. It usually occurs during childbearing years, but seems to be occurring increasingly during the teen years. Many patients with fibrositis say their pains are worse during cool, damp weather, or during periods of overexertion, anxiety and emotional stress. Symptoms in some women worsen during pregnancy and then are relieved after the delivery of the baby.

Infection seems to make fibrositis worse. Stress also plays a major role in the disease.

For many individuals, improvements often occur during warmer weather, vacations and relaxed activity. Better sleep, mild exercise and better management of stress help many people.

Bursitis

A condition frequently confused with arthritis is bursitis. Bursitis means a painful inflammation of the bursa, which are small, fluid-filled sacs near joints between muscles, bones ligaments, and tendons. Their function is to reduce friction and help absorb shocks.

Bursitis differs from arthritis in that inflammation involves the areas surrounding the joint rather than the joint itself. There are many varieties of bursitis, many of which are known by popular names. For example, prepatellar bursitis, known as housemaid's knees, is caused by prolonged kneeling on a hard surface, and frozen shoulder, which is the end result of an untreated form of bursitis of the shoulder.

Treatment for bursitis usually consists of anti-inflammatory medications and rest. Injections with steroids are helpful in some cases; physical therapy is also helpful. Application of an icepack may relieve pain for some individuals. In many cases, bursitis lasts only a short time.

In rare cases, a bursectomy — i.e., an operation to remove the bursa — may be performed.

41

Tennis/Golfer's Elbow

Tennis/golfer's elbow—technically known as lateral/medical epicondylitis — occurs in many people who overuse their arms during athletics, gardening, or other activities. Although the pain may feel similar to arthritis, this conditions is not arthritis. sufferers may experience pain during handshaking and lifting light-weight items. The condition consists of inflammation, degeneration of the common extensor tendon, and sometimes may involve tendon tears.

Treatment involves changing one's activities and preventing overuse of the forearm muscles. Ice packs, heat and NSAIDs help many people. For details see Chapter 4. Some individuals use a forearm brace, while others find that a local steroid injection at the tender spot in the elbow produces relief.

Frozen Shoulder

Frozen shoulder—technically known as pericapsulitis or adhesive capsulitis— causes general pain and tenderness as well as loss of motion. Frozen shoulder usually occurs after the age of 40 and often as a secondary problem after a fall or with another type of shoulder condition, diabetes, or inflammatory arthritis.

The conditions involves the adherence of the shoulder joint capsule to part of the neck, with the underarm muscles binding to themselves, causing a thickening and contraction or frozen feeling.

Diagnosis is made through arthrography, magnetic resonance imaging or MRI; or arthroscopy. For details see Chapter 3. Frozen shoulder is often treated in many different ways, including physical therapy, ice packs, ultrasound, gentle range of motion exercises, NSAIDs, corticosteroid injections, and surgery.

Housemaid's Knee

Housemaid's knee—technically known as prepatellar bursitis— may result from frequent kneeling. There may be pain and swelling of the knees, as well and increased tenderness.

Treatment may involve avoiding kneeling, heat, ice packs, rest, and gentle exercise.

Baker's Cyst

Baker's cyst—technically known as popliteal cysts—involves a swelling of the knee with mild or no discomfort initially. However, with full flexion of the knee, the individual experiences greater discomfort.

The condition involves a collection of fluid between the knee joint and the bursa. Popliteal cyst sometimes occur after reheumatoid arthritis, osteoarthritis, or injury to the knee. An arthrogram and ultrasound help a physician make a diagnosis. For details see Chapter 3.

Treatment may include injection of corticosteroids into the knee joint and in some cases into the cyst itself. When the cyst results from degenerative arthritis or an internal injury to the knee, surgical repair may become necessary.

Achilles Tendinitis

This condition may occur as a result of athletic overactivity, injury, or even improperly fitting shoes with a stiff heel counter. It may also develop along with inflammatory conditions such as ankylosing spondylitis, Reiter's syndrome, gout, or rheumatoid arthritis.

Achilles tendinitis involves pain, swelling and tenderness over the Achilles tendon at its attachment and near the attachment. Treatment includes rest, shoe correction, heel lift, gentle stretching, sometimes a splint, and in some cases, NSAIDs For details see Chapter 4. Generally, the tendon should not be injected with a corticosteroid, as it is subject to rupture.

Tenosynovitis

Inflammation of synovium of the tendon sheaths occurs in a wide variety of conditions of over-use particularly involving tendons of the thumb. This either blocks complete or partial movement of the thumb and causes pain. Drug treatment has little part to play in the management of the condition. Local corticosteriod injections are sometimes effective.

Muscle Pains

The medical term for muscle pain is myalgia. Myalgia occurs in many rheumatic disorders, including rheumatoid arthritis, systemic lupus erythematosus, and polymyalgia rheumatica and fibromyalgia.

Polymyalgia Rheumatica

This is a relatively rare condition of older people, usually not occurring before the age of 50. There is stiffness in the muscles of the hips, thighs, shoulders, and neck, as well as pain, particularly in the morning, making movement difficult.

Although the cause is unknown, it is often associated with rheumatoid arthritis, systemic lupus erythematosus (SLE), temporal arteritis, and cancer. The disorder affects more women then men.

Diagnosis, although difficult to confirm, is based on a physical examination, the patient's history, and blood tests. Treatment sometimes includes small doses of corticosteroid drugs.

Growing Pains

Many children, particularly age six through 12, experience vague aches and pains in their arms and legs, often at night for unknown reasons. Such aches may occasionally interfere with a child's sleep, but require no treatment. However, if there is swelling of joints, a physician should be consulted.

Collagen Vascular Diseases

There is a group of connective tissue diseases that are caused by malfunctioning of the immune system, often affecting blood vessels and producing secondary damage in the connective tissues. Included in the category of collagen vascular diseases are rheumatoid arthritis, systemic lupus erythematosus, scleroderma, and other less clearly defined disorders.

Scleroderma

Scleroderma is a disease of the connective tissue and may also affect the joints, skin, blood vessels, and internal organs such as the lungs and kidneys. The word scleroderma means *hard skin*; most people with this condition develop stiffness and tightness of their skin over their face, arms, and fingers.

The disease usually starts between age 30 and 50, and affects more women than men.

A frequent first symptom of scleroderma is an extreme sensitivity to cold in the fingers, resulting in tingling or numbness known as Raynaud's phenomenon. Swelling, a feeling of heat and tenderness are not as apparent in scleroderma as in rheumatoid arthritis. However, individuals who have scleroderma have a swelling of the tissue around the joints in the hands or feet and muscle weakness.

Causes of scleroderma are unknown. It is not contagious or inherited. Treatment is usually tailored to the individual case, and may involve use of medications, massage, careful choice of wearing apparel, quitting smoking, biofeedback training, and sleeping with the head of the bed raised to relieve digestive problems.

Dengue

This disease gives rise to a very acute form of peri-arthritis (that is, inflammation of surrounding tissues of a joint). Intense pain and sometimes swelling occur in the tendons and muscles around the joints. These usually disappear when the fever subsides, but may recur in the stage of convalescence and last for weeks or months. The condition should be differentiated from rheumatic fever, from which it differs in being epidemic and in not responding to salicylates. Pain killers are given to relieve pain.

Predisposing Factors of Arthritic Diseases

1. Normal ageing process is one of the likely factors for causing lack of elasticity and flexibility of cartilage in the joints due to wear and tear of the joint bone. This often leads to arthritic condition.

2. Over-straining the back may cause damage to ligaments and other vertebral discs.

3. Hereditary factor cannot be ruled out. Incidence of rheumatoid arthritis is higher than expected in twins and first degree relations.

4. Occupation and lifestyle may also be related to arthritis. For example, a particular kind of posture or strain on a particular joint may cause osteoarthrits of that part of the joint.

5. Overweight may also affects the larger weight-bearing joints — chiefly the hips, knees or spine of older people in osteoarthritis.

6. The manifestations of SLE (systemic lupus erythematosus) may become worse during pregnancy.

7. Rise in uric acid in blood serum is likely to cause gout.

8. Mental tension/stress cannot be ruled out for the emotional and physical manifestation of the disease, pain and depression.

9. Acute or chronic arthritis can occur when bacteria get into the joints.

10. Weather conditions have also been considered responsible for arthritis and gout. Damp and cold weather often causes and aggravates these conditions than dry and hot weather.

3

Diagnosing Arthritis

Just as no two fingerprints are indentical, no two cases of arthritis are exactly the same. Your physician's careful examination and studies will be important to your diagnosis, judging the results of therapy, and planning an ongoing treatment program that may include use of drugs, adequate rest, exercise, physical therapy, and a good, well-balanced diet, possibly surgery too. You will read about how these aspects of treatment may interact to help you to better health in the following chapters.

Investigations to Establish Arthritis

Blood Tests — What they tell: Physicians use several blood tests to help them diagnose some types of arthritis, particularly rheumatoid arthritis, gout and systemic lupus erythematosus (SLE). However, while blood tests are helpful, they are not diagnostic in rheumatological diseases.

Erythrocyte sedimentation rate (ESR): This test measures how fast red blood fall or form a sediment at the bottom of a glass tube full of whole blood when allowed to remain still for an hour. Individuals who have inflammation due to arthritis usually have higher sedimentation rates than others. The normal sedimentation rate is 0 to 6 mm at the end of one hour, based on Westegren Method. Upon improvement, the sedimentation rate usually decreases.

Antibody Tests: Antibodies are special kind of blood proteins to attach the antigens and render them harmless. Some abnormal antibodies—which causes harm to body cells—in the blood may suggest certain forms of arthritis. For example, persons who have rheumatoid arthritis usually have large amounts of a substance called rheumatoid factor (RF) in their blood, which is not present in a normal, healthy body. Thus the test known as the rheumatoid factor (RF) test or RA latex test helps physicians diagnose rheumatoid arthritis.

Another test for abnormal antibodies is the antinuclear antibody test (ANA), which detects a group of auto antibodies in the blood serum that are found in people who have lupus and scleroderma and in some people who have rheumatoid arthritis. For details see Chapter 2. One antinuclear antibody, known as anti-DNA, is particularly useful in diagnosing lupus.

Complement Test: The complement test measures the amount of complement — a substance in normal serum that is destructive to bacteria and other cells in the blood. In simple terms, *complement* involves a group of blood substances that help antibodies fight disease-causing agents that enter the body by promoting inflammation. Some people who have active lupus often have lower than normal amounts of complement. For details see Chapter 2.

Uric Acid Test: The uric acid tests measures the amount of uric acid in the blood. People who have gout usually have elevated levels of uric acid (hyperuricemia). The normal level is 3.0 to 6.0 mg/100 ml in blood serum.

Urine Tests: Urine tests (urinalysis) show whether the urine contains red blood cells, protein, or a variety of abnormal substances which are normally not present in a healthy body. Detection of these substances may help the physician diagnose kidney damage in certain rheumatic diseases, such as lupus, as well as the side effects of some drugs used in treating arthritis.

Radiography as a Diagnostic Tool

Magnetic Resonance Imaging (MRI): MRI is a diagnostic technique that helps the physician diagnose arthritis by showing cross-sectional images of structures and organs in the body without using X-ray or other radiation. The technique is useful for examining areas in the musculoskeletal system, lumbar spine. cervical spine, knees and shoulders.

MRI has been in use since the early 1980s. The patient, in a lying down position, is surrounded by electromagnets and exposed to short bursts of magnetic fields and radio waves; the bursts stimulate atoms in the patient's tissues to emit signals which are detected and analyzed by computer to create an image of a slice of the patient's body. A computer linked to the MRI scanner creates an image of the area being scanned and displays it on a monitor for viewing by the diagnostician.

MRI is usually an outpatient procedure and the scan usually takes about half an hour.

X-rays: In some fairly advanced cases of arthritis, X-rays may be useful in making a diagnosis. In early cases, the bones and cartilage are not damaged enough to show changes on X-rays. However, X-rays taken early in the course of disease may be useful to detect changes and progression of the disease when compared with later X-rays.

X-rays are also useful to determine how well certain treatments are working to control bone damage and to determine if people need joint surgery.

X-rays are particularly useful for identifying ankylosing spondylitis for finding bone growths called osteophytes in people who have osteoarthritis, and for finding crystals that cause a disease sometimes called pseudogout—also known as calcium pyrophosphate dihydeate crystal deposition disease or CPPD disease. For details see Chapter 2.

A myelogram is a type of X-ray used to find spinal disc problems that may cause back pain. After injecting a dye into the spinal canal, X-rays are taken to determine if bulging discs are pressing on nerves. Computerized axial tomography (CAT scan) permits this diagnosis to be made in some people without a myelogram.

Computerized axial tomography (CAT scan) is a special

form of X-ray, helpful in determining arthritis in the cervical and lumbar spine (neck and lower back). The scan enables physicians to see if the patient has any herniated discs or impingement on the spinal cord by the bone spurs. This technique has been available since the middle 1970s.

Arthrography is another procedure in which a special dye in injected to coat the cartilage before an X-ray is taken. The joint cavity thus can be seen by the physician and any damage to the cartilage surface can be determined. This procedure is not as widely used since the development of MRI.

Examination of Synovial Fluid: It can be of great value when the diagnosis is in doubt. Infection is excluded or detected by microscopic examination of a Gram stained smear and culture for bacterial products. In inflammetory joints disease the synovial fluid is of low viscosity, turbid, clots on standing and contains many cells.

4

Treatments for Arthritis

Medical historians know that many people have had arthritis since the earliest recorded history. Treatments have been sought and tried, and many claims for cures have been made. Arthritis treatments range from highly priced quack remedies to modern drugs that help millions of people.

Treatments for arthritis include a good, well-balanced diet, rest, exercise, heat, and possibly surgery. For more information on surgical techniques to relieve painful arthritis, please refer to Chapter 5. Rest, exercise therapy, and diet are covered in Chapters 6 and 7.

HOME COMFORTS

Many people try traditional home remedies before seeking medical attention for various aches and pains, Indeed, some home remedies help many people, and may offer temporary relief. However, if symptoms do not improve with simple remedies, medical attention should be sought.

Heat Treatments: Hot Baths, Hot Compresses

Heat is relaxing and soothing. It can help your joints move better with less pain by relaxing painfully tight muscles. Various forms of heat are frequently advised. These include hot baths, hot packs, heat lamps, and paraffin wax applications. A hot bath first thing in the morning may provide a better start to your day. Occasionally however, some people respond better to cold packs around an acutely inflamed joint than to heat.

Heat can be applied in many different ways. Many people find that hot baths reduce stiffness, and warm pools are helpful when their range of motion is limited; the buoyancy of the water enables them to perform movements they cannot do out of water. Many individuals find that water exercise programs are especially beneficial. Hot compresses can be prepared by soaking towels in hot water, wringing them out, and applying to the painful area.

Electric heating pads may be placed on the painful area for short periods of time. However, care must be taken to be sure the appliance is in good condition and is used appropriately.

Cold Treatments

For some arthritic pains, cold treatment helps provide relief. An easy way to make a cold compress is by filling a plastic bag with ice cubes. Place a towel over the skin, and the ice bag above the towel. Also, a towel can be soaked in ice water, wrung out, and placed on the painful area. A dry towel or piece of plastic wrap should be placed between the cold compress and the skin to protect the skin from effects of the cold compress.

Some individuals find that alternating between heat and cold provides some relief. This is easier to do for hands and feet than other areas of the body, as hands and feet can be soaked alternatley in hot or cold water. Usually, cold treatments are recommended for the first 24 to 48 hours after an acute injury.

Massage

Massage relieves tension and provides relaxation to the affected area. Deep kneading or gentle circular motions may be appropriate for different individuals and for different types of aches. For some areas of the body such as hands, knees, feet and neck, self-massage may be possible; for other areas, assistance of a partner or professional masseur may be necessary.

Pain Control: Electrical Stimulation

A recent advance in relieving or controlling pain is the transcutaneous electrical nerve stimulator (TENS). When the individual wearing the TENS unit turns it on, a low level of electricity is applied to designated areas of the body, sometimes producing a tingling sensation. The unit may be kept on a few minutes or a few hours, according to the needs of the individual. The size of the TENS units ranges from about the size of a package of cigarettes to larger devices used in medical centres.

PHYSICAL THERAPY

Physical therapy is often recommended in addition to exercises you can do at home. Some people need ongoing physical therapy, while others do well with an occasional series of therapy treatments, which are then followed by an at-home routine. You may be advised to have your therapy at a local hospital or health centre or have a therapist visit you at home.

While medication may seem to be the most dramatic form of arthritis treatment, most physicians say that it is the interaction of the drugs and what the patient does for himelf or herself that actually brings about the most relief from arthritis. Medication without exercise isn't as effective.

In all cases of arthritis, a comprehensive programme of medication, balanced exercise and rest, and a nutritious diet provides the best change for relief of pain, prevention of deformity, and restoration of a normal life.

The treatment of arthritis consists of many parts. Physicians agree that the most important part is what you can do for yourself. How you integrate the professional recommendations with your lifestyle can make a difference in how you feel.

Importance of Professional Guidance

To be sure that the treatment you take for your arthritis is a tried and proven one, follow your physician's advice. The many available methods of treatment can be confusing. Self-diagnosis and self-treatment aren't advised by the reputable medical community. Your physician will decide whether or not you have arthritis, and if you do, what treatment, or combination of treatments, will be most likely to help you. Advertising today sometimes makes it look as if one could easily purchase over-the-counter drugs to treat arthritis. While some remedies may provide some relief for some people, using a non-prescription therapy may only put off beginning a more effective therapy that will bring about more long-range improvements. While physcans do prescribe medications, they also coordinate interdisciplinary services aimed at improving your overall health, your nutrition, your body's flexibility, and guidance on how you can help yourself.

How can you recognize an undesirable arthritis clinic or health care centre? The best single way to identify such places is that they all promise a cure. Reputable physicians and insititutions don't promise a cure. They do promise, however, to try to determine the cause of a pain and to try treatment which they know has been reasonably effective in similar cases. Physicians also warn against any health centre that uses the same *miracle treatment* to cure *all* types of pain, since arthritis is an individual disease and treatment for each case must be individualized. Today many medications are available to your physician for inclusion in your arthritis treatment. The medications have been known to help others, and some of them may help you.

DRUGS

There are many approved drugs from which your physician can choose. Aspirin is the most commonly prescribed drug. There are also alternatives to aspirin, known as nonsteroidal antiinflammatory drugs (NSAIDs), as well as gold salts, penicillamine, antimalarials, painkillers, uric acid-lowering drugs, steroids, and experimental drugs that are used only in some research centres.

Aspirin

Aspirin is the first-choice drug for arthritis because it acts both as an analgesic (painkiller) and in higher doses as an antiinflammatory agent. As a painkiller, aspirin acts on the central nervous system to reduce the ability to feel pain. As an antiinflammatory agent it must be taken in specific dosages as recommended by your physician. To explain the antiinflammatory process of aspirin, the US Arthritis Foundation says, "Aspirin stops the production of prostaglandins, substances released at the site of inflammation which apparently increase pain by sensitizing nerve endings. By interfering with prostaglandin production, the drug blocks pain and reduces inflammation... To take full advantage of aspirin's anti-inflammatory powers, a person with arthritis may have to take as many as 15 to 20 tablets per day."

Many people are impressed with drugs that have complicated technical names. They find it difficult to believe that a simple non-prescription remedy, taken under a physician's guidance, can do much for serious ailments such as arthritis. Although aspirin is a non-prescription drug, it is not recommended that arthritis sufferers take large quantities of aspirin without direction from a physician. Each individual case of arthritis is different, and each person reacts in different ways to the action of aspirin. Your physician knows you best and knows what is most likely to help you. If your doctor has started you on an aspirin programme, be sure to take the prescribed amount of aspirin. Although you may feel better on some days, do not stop taking the aspirin; the antiinflammatory power of the drug will be reduced greatly if you stop taking it. Like many drugs, it must be taken steadily or it will not work properly. Also, once you begin taking high doses of aspirin, it may be several days to a week before you start to feel its full effects.

If you are on aspirin therapy, many physicians advise buying large bottles of an unadvertised brand, such as generic aspirin; otherwise, rather than higher quality, you will be paying for the advertising costs.

Should you notice any unpleasant side effects from your aspirin dosage, call your physician. You may be advised to change your dosage. Within a short time after you decrease the dosage your side effect symptoms will probably go away.

If aspirin is so effective in treating arthritis, why don't more people take it? Some people cannot take aspirin because it upsets their stomach. For this reason some favour buffered aspirin, aspirin mixed with antacids, or coated aspirin. These types of aspirin may cause less indigestion. Other people have conditions in which complications might arise if they took aspirin, such as those who have peptic ulcers. Fortunately, there are aspirin alternatives, as described below, for people who cannot tolerate aspirin. They work in much the same way as aspirin.

Painkillers

Drugs that relieve pain are often used in the treatment of arthritis. Although they may provide some temporary relief, they do not actually help the arthritis. Instead, they cover it up, which can be dangerous because it often means that more effective treatment is postponed.

Painkillers such as acetaminophen, propoxyphene, oxycodone, demerol, and codeine are used in short-term treatment of arthritis pain. However, because arthritis is a chronic disease, most physicians advise that any drug on which the patient might become overly dependent should be avoided. Although these drugs may be prescribed in special circumstances, they are rarely used in the long-term treatment of arthritis.

Nonsteroidal Anti-Inflammatory Drugs (NSAIDs)

These are aspirin substitutes. The nonsteroidal aspect of these drugs is important. Steroids have serious side effects and usually are tried only after other drugs have proved to be ineffective.

Most of the NSAIDs act like aspirin in that they interfere with the formation of prostaglandins, which trigger inlfammation. Also like aspirin, these aspirin substitutes usually must be taken several times a day. Researchers are working on perfecting NSAIDs that can be taken in single daily doses.

Some of the more widely used NSAIDs are sold under the generic names of indomethacin, phenylbutazone, naproxen, sulindac, fenoprofen, ibuprofen, tolmetin, meclofenemate, and piroxicam. These drugs are not without side effects, however. Some people using them have noticed dizziness, headache, stomach upset, fluid retention, nausea, diarrhea, constipation, itching and ringing in the ears. Whenever you notice any side effect while taking medication, call your doctor. You may be advised to live with the side effect becaue it will subside after a while. However, your physician may determine whether the side effect may be harmful to you and change your medication.

Steroids

Steroids are the most potent anti-inflammatory drugs available. They can rapidly reduce pain and inflammation. But they must be used under a physician's careful supervision because they can cause numerous serious side effects if taken in high daily doses for more than a two-month period.

According to the US Arthritis Foundation, steroids taken orally, while still useful in special situations, are being prescribed less often by specialists in the treatment of rheumatoid arthritis. Direct injection of steroids into a particularly painful joint, on the other hand, is still an effective technique for providing temporary relief without the side effects of steroids taken orally.

Normally, your body makes its own steroids, but when you begin taking steroids as drugs your body slowly loses its ability to produce them. For this reason, when you go off a steroid programme, you must do it very slowly so your body can regain its ability to produce its own steroids. An abrupt cessation of the drug could subject your body to a harmful jolt. This is why it is most important to follow your doctor's exact instructions concerning steroids.

Unless they are given in very small doses, steroids taken orally on a daily basis will eventually cause serious side effects in all patients. The side effects of steroids most often appear from several weeks to one year after a person begins taking the drug in moderate to high doses. They can include ulcers, profound mental changes, high blood pressure, a high propensity for bruising, weight gain, and weakening of the muscles. Over longer periods of time the bones become more brittle, the skin becomes thin and cataracts may develop. Steroid users may also become psychologically dependent on them, making it difficult to stop taking steroids in spite of the doctor's orders.

While steroids are usually taken by mouth or given by injection into the painful area, a third, less effective method is injection of ACTH, adrenocorticotropic hormone. This hormone stimulates the body's own adrenal glands to produce more steroids.

Of all the steroids, prednisone is the most common and the least expensive. Other steroids frequently prescribed are known by these generic names: prednisolone, methylprednisolone, triamcinolone, and dexamethasone.

Remission-Inducing Drugs

Gold salts, antimalarial drugs, and penicillamine are frequently used to treat rheumatoid arthritis. These medications have a unique ability to produce a drug-induced remission of disease in some patients with rheumatoid arthritis. While they are not antiinflammatory drugs, the symptoms of arthritis usually improve when these drugs produce a remission of the inflammation and destruction of the joints.

Gold Salts: Gold treatment given by weekly injections has been used for the treatment of rheumatoid arthritis for about 50 years. For a long time doctors were not sure how well gold salts worked, but recently gold has been found effective in many, but not all, of the cases of rheumatoid arthritis that are resistant to other treatments. It may take as long as several months of injections to find out if gold salts work for a patient.

Still in the experimental stage is a new gold-containing drug that can be taken orally. This would be a great advantage, because the present weekly injections may be painful and require frequent visits to the physician's office.

Antimalarial Drugs: Antimalarial drugs such as chloroquine and hydroxychloroquine sulphate are often used in the treatment of rheumatoid arthritis, though it is not known exactly how they work. They have been helpful for many people when taken in limited doses over a long period of time. Most people tolerate them well, though side effects sometimes occur. Since loss of vision is the most worrisome side effect of antimalarial drugs, frequent eye examinations by an ophthalmologist are required while taking these drugs.

Penicillamine: Not to be confused with the related compound penicillin, this recently released drug, like gold, is reserved for persons with severe rheumatoid arthritis that does not respond well to other therapies. People who are allergic to penicillin may still take penicillamine safely.

Penicillamine may work extremely well for one patient and not at all for another. Also like gold, penicillamine must be taken for several months as a test to find out if it works for the individual.

Cytotoxic Drugs

While cytotoxic drugs are usually used to treat people who have cancer or have received organ transplants, they are also used for some individuals who have severe arthritis. These drugs work by suppressing the immune system and thereby block the actions of cells that create the abnormal antibodies in autoimmune diseases and of those that are involved in inflammation. However, because cytotoxic drugs are very potent and have serious side effects, physicians use them only in cases where other drugs have not been effective. The most frequently used cytotoxic drugs are cyclophosphamide and azathioprine (generic names).

Methotrexate, a drug used to treat cancer, is also becoming more widely used to treat rheumatoid arthritis, psoriatic arthritis, and in certain situations, in connective tissue diseases.

5

Surgical Treatment for Arthritis

You may have heard dramatic stories abut improvements made in arthritic conditions by joint replacement operations and other surgical techniques. There have been many success stories in recent years. Surgical techniques are effective in many cases, but before you begin thinking about replacement of your aching joints or a mechanical repair of them, arthritis experts recommend exhausting all other therapies first. In most cases surgery is advised only after other techniques, such as drug therapy, rest, physical therapy, exercise, and improvement of overall health, have been tried and have failed to produce good results.

Joint surgery for arthritis requires expertise and should be performed in specialized facilities that also can offer other forms of treatment, such as rehabilitation therapy. If you are advised a surgical procedure, you may want to obtain a second opinion and thoroughly check out the surgeon who is suggested to perform surgery as well as the facility at which it will be performed.

Since the 1960s, when the first successful total hip-joint replacement operation was performed, there have been many advances in surgical techniques to relieve the chronic pain and permanent disability of arthritis. The first total hip replacement utilized a joint consisting of metal and plastic parts and was the result of a collaborative effort among engineers, orthopaedic surgeons, and arthritis specialists.

As a result of success with hip joint replacement, researchers have developed techniques to improve other joints. Artificial components can now replace the knee joint. Other surgical techniques have been improved for use on the ankle, shoulder, elbow, wrist and hand.

Is surgery for You?

Can surgery help you? Have you asked your physician about the possibilities of correcting your joint defects through surgical procedures ? Has your physican recommended surgery ? Before advising surgery your surgeon will assess the potential for improvement in pain and restoration of movement that you can expect after the suggested surgical procedure. The outlook for improvement will depend largely on how severely your joints and tendons are damaged or pulled out of place, the general condition of your health, and how well you follow recommendations for exercise and physical therapy during the recovery period.

You and your physician will want to be realistic in your expectation of what surgery can do for you. If you have a severe deformity of a joint, you can usually expect some improvement in the range of motion and relief of pain. However, you should not expect your joint to have the same range of motion it had before your disease developed. Your physician, surgeon, and physical therapist will review these possibilities with you before you make your decision.

Your physician or surgeon may have reasons for advising against a surgical correction. Your overall health is a major consideration. If you have any chronic conditions, surgery may be postponed until the other conditions have cleared up. For example, if your have a bacterial infection, such as bronchitis or a bladder infection, the infection might spread to the area operated on after surgery.

All surgical procedures are a severe strain on the body. if you have any problems with breathing or your heart, joint surgery may not be advised for you because the procedures involved in the surgery may place an additional burden on your respiratory and cardiovascular systems.

Another reason for advising against arthritis surgery or postponing it, is obesity. If you are heavier than your ideal weight, the extra kilograms put extra stress on your heart, lungs, and weight-bearing joints. The outlook for your recovery after joint surgery is not as favourable. The excess weight puts added strain on the joint and may pose problems in doing the rehabilitation exercises for strengthening the new joint after surgery.

If you and your physician decide that a surgical procedure may provide some relief and improvement, the real outcome will depend on what you do for yourself. You will want to take an active part in following recommendations regarding medication, joint protection, rest and exercise. Ask about the kinds of routines that will be recommended for your post-operative recovery and rehabilitation. Be sure that you will be able to carry out the prescribed programmes before you undertake the expense and discomfort associated with surgery.

Following are the terms most frequently used in discussing surgical possibilities for treating arthritis. An understanding of these terms will help you in planning your arthritis treatment with your physician.

Terms Used in Joint Surgery

Arthodesis: Also known as *bone fusion,* this is done most commonly in the ankles and wrists to relieve pain. When these joints are fused, or *frozen,* they are not flexible but are without pain.

Arthroplasty: Joints are rebuilt using this technique. It involves resurfacing or relining the ends of bones where the cartilage has worn away and destruction of the bone has occurred. The term also refers to replacement with a prosthesis (artificial part) of the entire joint. Results of total joint replacement have been good. A better understanding of joint replacement, joint function, improved materials, and surgical methods has benefited many people who were disabled by pain and loss of mobility.

Arthroscopy : This technique involves visualizing the inside of joints by looking through a thin instrument resembling a drinking straw called an *arthroscope,* which is inserted through a 6mm incision. Once an abnormality is seen it can frequently be repaired with special surgical instruments inserted through another small incision. Arthroscopy may be performed under local anaesthesia, often on an outpatient basis, with fewer side effects and a shorter rehabilitation period than associated with arthrotomy.

Arthrotomy: The procedure during which joints are surgically opened to allow accurate diagnosis and make surgical repairs is known as arthrotomy. This procedure is being done less and less with the advent of arthroscopy.

Cartilage: The covering of the ends of the bones. The cartilage becomes frayed and pitted in osteoarthritis, interfering with smooth movement of the joint. This wear and tear on cartilage on weight-bearing joints such as the hip or knee contributes to pain, deformity and loss of mobility. In the fingers, the condition causes stiffness and a knobby look.

Joint Synovium: The place in the body where two bones join together—the tissue lining the joints. The inflammation in the synovium in rheumatoid arthritis causes the tissue to enlarge or thicken, damaging the cartilage and bone nearby. Such inflammation causes swelling and pain.

Osteotomy: This operation is performed to correct bone deformities or improper alignment of a bone. The surgeon cuts and resets the bone, permitting it to heal in a better position.

Resection: This is the removal of a bone or part of a bone. This technique is used when the metatarsal joints of the feet make walking painful and difficult. Painful bunions are also removed by resection.

Synovectomy: This type of surgery involves opening the joint and removing the membrane that is inflamed by arthritis.

Frequently, however, the synovial membrane grows back and becomes inflamed again.

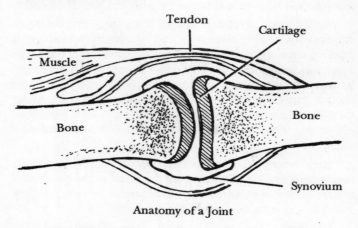

Anatomy of a Joint

Surgical Techniques

While several types of techniques are commonly used, each case must be considered individually. What is appropriate for one person may not be appropriate for another.

Synovectomy is one of the oldest surgical procedures to relieve pain in joints and has been done for more than 50 years. This procedure involves removing the inner lining of a joint that has become thickened and painful. It has been performed most often on the knee, wrist, and fingers. A disadvantage of this operation is that in many cases, the synovial membrane grows back and symptoms may return.

Tendon repair is frequently done to improve the disability of rheumatoid arthritis in the fingers and hand when the disease destroys the tendon or causes the outer surface of the bone to fray and tear the tendon sheath. Such procedures may involve removing the damaged bone surface, repairing worn tissue, and securing weakened tissue to healthy tissue nearby.

Total replacement of the hip and knee joints has become fairly common and has a good rate of success.

Surgical Benefits for Specific Joints

Hip: The greatest success with joint surgery for arthritis thus far has been through replacement of hip joints. According to the US Arthritis Foundation, more than 75,000 such replacements are performed each year. The success rate for osteoarthritis is 95 percent and is almost as high for rheumatoid arthritis.

Two types of techniques are used. One is total hip replacement, and the other is resurfacing. In deciding which procedure is most appropriate and will be most successful for the individual patient, the surgeon will consider the age of the patient and the condition of the bones. Until the past few years, bone cement used in total hip replacement had poor holding power and that operation was reserved for older people. Now, with improvements in the cement used, expectations are that the cement will hold for about 25 years, and hip replacement operations are now being done for younger people.

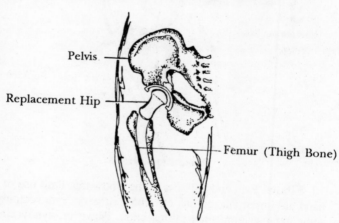

Pelvis

Replacement Hip

Femur (Thigh Bone)

Total Hip Joint Replacement

The other technique, resurfacing, involves cleaning away the top of the thigh bone (femur) and capping it with a metal covering. The socket of the hip is also cleaned and lined with a plastic material. Although this procedure has the same pain-relieving and motion-restoring potential as total replacement, it is not known whether this procedure will last as long as total joint replacement. However, should it be required, a total replacement can be done later on.

Knee: The major surgical procedures to improve the function of the knee joints are arthroscopy and partial or total joint replacement. These techniques offer relief from the serious problems of pain, instability, and loss of mobility but do not always restore full function in terms of flexibility and weight bearing. About 30,000 knee replacements are performed each year in the US.

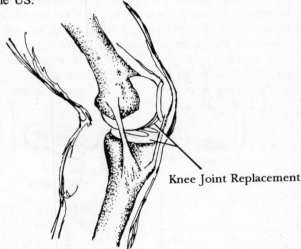

Knee Joint Replacement

Knee Replacement

Elbow: Pain and stiffness in the elbow that limit use of the hand are important reasons for elbow surgery. Synovectomy is sometimes accompanied by resection. However, synovectomy does not help if there is osteoarthritis in the elbow or if the problem has been caused by injury. Sometimes physicians will recommend resurfacing or joint replacement instead.

Shoulder: Pain in the shoulder can sometimes be helped by arthroscopy. Total joint replacement also relieves the pain in some cases but usually restores only a limited range of motion. Shoulder joint replacement requires a post-operative period of many months for recovery.

Ankle and Foot: Surgical procedures are performed in many joints in the foot to correct defects caused by arthritis. Arthrodesis, or fusion of the bone of the foot or ankle, is a commonly performed operation. Replacement of the ankle also is done under some circumstances. When the metatarsal arch is painful and prevents walking, resection of the heads of the metatarsals may be considered. With resection toe deformities can be corrected for some individuals.

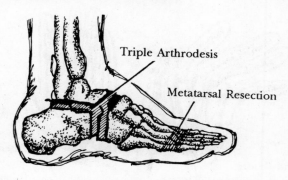

Triple Arthrodesis

Metatarsal Resection

Sites of Two Types of Foot Surgery

Hand and Wrist: Several types of surgical procedures are done on the hands and wrists to restore function after they have been damaged by arthritis. One type of surgery is aimed at the improvement of a condition called *dorsal tenosynovitis*, which affects the lining of the long tendons on the back of the hand. Sometimes the affected tendon tears apart and requires repair. If this occurs, surgical repair of these ruptured tendons gives good results for the majority of patients and recovery is fairly the rapid. Synovectomy, done for both the fingers and the wrists in early stages of deformity, has not been successful. The dexterity of the fingers and hand is sometimes improved by operations done to tighten or loosen the pull of the tendons.

Another technique used to relieve the crippling effects of

arthritis in the fingers involves silicone rubber implants in the finger joints. This is appropriate in some cases and requires careful analysis by the surgeon before a decision regarding the surgery is made.

Several techniques are also available for the wrist. Arthrodesis can relieve pain and provide more stability for the hand, but some limited motion will result. The range of motion may be improved with resection of the end of one of the bones in the wrist. Another possibility, in some cases, is total joint replacement.

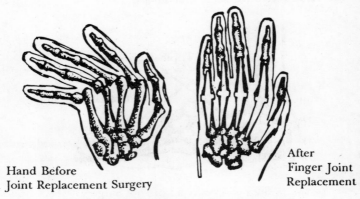

Hand Before
Joint Replacement Surgery

After
Finger Joint
Replacement

Finger Joint Replacement

What to Expect After Surgery

Before you agree to have surgery to relieve your pain or correct your deformity caused by arthritis, be sure to plan ahead so that your recovery period can be as effective as possible. For example, you may want to make arrangements to have some help at home or to stay where someone can help you during the first weeks after surgery. You may need a period of rest and some time to get used to certain aids, such as splints, crutches, or a cane while you are recovering. You will have an exercise routine to do at home as well as physical therapy at your health centre. It will take at least a few weeks, or longer after some procedures, for you to resume your usual routine.

What to Ask Your Doctor about Surgical Procedures

When considering surgery you will want to review many important questions. Generally, they should be discussed with your physician. Here are some questions to ask your doctor:*

- ☐ What other kinds of treatment is available other than surgery?
- ☐ Can you explain the surgical procedure?
- ☐ How long will the surgery take?
- ☐ What, if any, risks are involved?
- ☐ Will I need a blood transfusion?
- ☐ What type of anaesthesia will I have?
- ☐ How much improvement can I expect from this procedure?
- ☐ Will other surgery be necessary?
- ☐ If surgery is chosen, how will my family doctor be involved in my hospitalization?
- ☐ How often have you performed this type of surgery?
- ☐ May I speak with a patient who has undergone this surgery?
- ☐ How long should I expect to stay in the hospital?
- ☐ Will I receive medication for pain?
- ☐ How long will I have to stay in bed after surgery?
- ☐ How long before physical therapy is started?
- ☐ What restrictions will be placed on my activities, such as driving, climbing stairs, bending, eating, making love?
- ☐ Will I need special equipment at home?

Surgical techniques have helped many people with arthritis. These techniques may help you. However, because each person's arthritis is an individual matter, your doctor and health care team can best evaluate whether or not surgical techniques will be appropriate for your case. If you do have surgery, however, your active participation during the recovery period in doing exercises and physical therapy will be an important key to the success of the procedures.

* Adapted from *Arthritis Surgery, Information to Consider*, Arthritis Foundation, 1981.

6

Rest, Exercise and Physical Therapy

For most individuals rest, exercise and physical therapy are important parts of treatment for arthritis. Rest helps reduce inflammation and muscle spasm, while exercise strengthens muscles and tendons and helps them to better support the joints.

Maintaining a proper balance between rest and exercise, and exercising properly are the keys to a successful arthritis exercise programme.

Rest

While rest can relieve the strain on affected joints, too much rest can cause further loss of use of joints and muscles. Your physician will help you work out a good balalnce between rest and exercise so that too much bed rest does not weaken you and too much exercise does not make you overly tired. Often, in cases of osteoarthritis, rest will be helpful at times when overuse of joints has caused discomfort. Also, joint pain due to arthritis can be relieved by techniques such as splinting by which the unintentional motion of an inflamed joint is limited, resulting in pain relief. Your physician and physical therapist can instruct you, if necessary, in the ways to rest particular joints.

Exercise

How much and what type of exercise you should do depends on which joints are affected, the kind of arthritis you have, how severe the pain or inflammation is, and your overall health. Some of the stiffness and weakness of arthritis can be relieved with mild exercise. For some individuals, maintaining joint mobility and muscle strength can help prevent some of the crippling deformities caused by arthritis.

Swimming is a good exercise for individuals with arthritis. Because approximately one-half of your body weight is supported by the water, it is easier to exercise and move in the water. It may give you a good feeling to move more normally while in the water. Many community centres and gyms now have water exercise and other special programmes for patients with arthritis. To find out about swimming activities for people with arthritis, call your local chapter of the Arthritis Foundation or check with your local community health centre or hospital.

Despite the presence of arthritis, you may continue to enjoy many forms of exercise, such as golf, tennis, boating, skating, skiing, or horseback riding. There may be times when you do not feel like participating, but being active when you can in a sport you enjoy will be helpful to you.

While the exercise you get in everyday living is helpful (such as doing housework or sports), there are exercises planned specifically for individuals with arthritis and specifically tailored for individual needs. Your personalized exerceise programme should include prescribed movements with specific purposes related to your joints and surrounding muscles.

Based on recommendations from the US Arthritis Foundation, the following are some helpful reminders about exercise:

1. Do your exercises on a regular basis. Do them on good days and bad, even if you have to modify your program because you are having a flare-up.

2. Make your exercises part of your daily life and do not skip them, even if you think they have become monotonous.

71

3. Be careful not to overdo. Too much exercise that aggravates your joints can be harmful. If increased pain in your joints lasts for several hours or extends into the next day, you may have done too much.

4. Learn to detect the difference between increased joint pain and muscle soreness after new exercises, which is a normal response to new activity.

5. Remember that your exercise needs may change with time to meet altered needs. Your physician and physical therapist will work closely with you to advise you of changes to make in your exercise routine.

6. Keep in mind that often it may be difficult to observe signs of improvement and that even a properly exercised joint may lose some motion during a flare-up of rheumatoid arthritis. However, joints that are not exercised on a regular basis may become more rapidly deformed than those that are.

7. Stick to your exercise programme in order to maximize your ability to maintain mobility and lead a normal life.

Benefits of Exercise: Use It or Lose It

There are numerous benefits of exercise. It leads to increased strength and flexibility in the muscles and ligaments surrounding the joints. In addition, it helps to maintain or increase the strength of bone. Exercises, such as swimming or walking, have beneficial effects on the heart that promote increased endurance and circulation and fight deterioration of the arteries.

Every tissue in the body requires certain foods or nutrients to work effectively. Most tissues have arteries that bring essential foods to them, but this is not true of the joint cartilage. It is only through movement that nourishment is brought by the synovial fluid to the joint cartilage and that waste products are removed. Thus, exercise promotes good joint nutrition.

Exercise is a way we can prevent the loss of function that may accompany arthritis. If you do not use a muscle or joint you will lose strength and mobility, and thus, function. Slow progress is to be expected, particularly if your arthritis is severe or your joint limitations have existed for a long time.

When Should You Exercise?

Exercise daily for the rest of your life. It is the *weekend warrior* who gets into trouble with painful strained muscles and ligaments. The only time a joint should not be exercised is when it is inflamed, or *hot* (swollen red, tender to the touch).

Find a specific time and place to exercise and make this a part of your daily routine. You will have to decide on the best time, but consider the following. It is best to exercise when, one you have the least pain, two you have the least stiffness, three you are not tired, and four your medication is having maximum effect. You probably want one such period early in the day, and one later.

What Can You Do to Prepare for Exercise?

Athletes learn that warming up before exercise means a more productive session. it helps prevent injuries. Here are some warm-up suggestions.

1. A slow general stretch: Lying in bed, a) stretch one arm up and then the other, b) push arms forward, opening hands wide, c) pull arms back and close hands, d) pull knees up and do a few bicycle turns in the air, e) stretch legs out straight, f) roll to the side, swinging legs off the edge of the bed, using momentum to help you sit up. This warm-up is helpful when first getting up in the morning and is very similar to what a cat does as it gets up from a rest.

2. Begin your exercise programme with small movements in a pain-free range.

3. Massage can be used to relax stiff joints and muscles prior to exercise. However, it is best not to massage deeply a hot joint.

4. Apply heat prior to exercise. Heat tends to relax joints and muscles and relieve pain. All of the following are acceptable ways of applying heat. a) Take a long, hot bath or shower. Aim the full force of the water at the painful joint(s). Hand-held

showers with a massage unit can be pleasant. Use caution and stand up slowly as the heat sometimes causes dizziness. b) An electric heating pad may be placed over the affected area. c) Fill a hot-water bottle with hot water. Be sure it is not hot enough to burn you. Again, it is best not to lie directly on the water bottle. d) Stand next to your heater or radiator.

5. If you don't get good results from heat, the application of cold may prove more effective, especially for the hot joint of rheumatoid arthritis. Cold relaxes muscles and produces a numbing effect, thus decreasing pain and increasing joint motion. As with heat, there are a few important principles of application: a) If you are especially sensitive to cold or have decreased sensation do not apply cold. Ask your doctor or therapist if you are unsure. b) Apply just long enough to achieve a numbing effect—no more than 15 to 20 minutes. c) Be cautious when exercising after applying cold; the numbing effect may allow you to overdo it. Remember, if the joint is hot. Restrict exercise to moving the joint through its full range of motion twice a day. d) Place the cold pack over the joint, not between the joint and a firm surface. e) Check during and after application for any sign of a break in the skin.

6. Cold packs can be bought, or you can create your own. Use whichever cold pack is easiest and most effective for you: a) Several resourceful people have suggested a sack of frozen peas! You can refreeze it and use it again. b) Massage with a large ice cube. c) Make a slush pack: Line a bowl with two heavy plastic bags; fill with three cups water and one cup denatured alcohol. Fasten the bags and place the bowl in the freezer until slush forms. You can refreeze a slush pack.

How Should You Exercise?

Be consistent and stick to your chosen set of exercise. Begin at a comfortable level and gradually increase the number of repetitions. Progress more slowly with rheumatoid joints that are prone to hot periods. With this gradual progression you will avoid unnecessary pain.

Exercises for arthritis should be performed with a slow, steady rhythm. Give your muscles time to relax between repetitions of each exercise (10 to 15 seconds).

It is important to coordinate your breathing with exercise. Breathe deeply and rhythmically as you exercise; never hold your breath. Interspersing deep breathing with exercise ensures an adequate oxygen supply to working muscles as well as release of tension. Deep breathing involves inhaling slowly and gently through your nose and drawing air down into your abdomen. Hold for at least five counts. Exhale slowly and gently through lightly closed lips for at least five counts. You can do this breating exercise in between the exercises described later.

What Should You Avoid?

Remember that your exercises should minimize stress on the joints. Avoid high-tension exercises such as weight lifting. If your weight-bearing joints (hips, knees, ankles, or spine) are affected, jogging should be approached cautiously. Bicycling for a painful knee should also be approached with caution: set a stationary bicycle on the lowest resistance.

If a chosen exercise for one joint places excessive stress on another involved joint—for example, a shoulder exercise that stresses an involved hand, or a hip exercise that stresses a painful low back—modify the exercise or substitute another.

As stated earlier, avoid exercising the hot, inflamed joint, but remember to move it through its full range of motion twice a day. Deep massage of the joint pain should also be avoided. Never take extra medication to mask joint pain before exercising.

Since warmth helps relax stiff muscles and joints, avoid becoming chilled during exercise. Wear warm clothing and do not exercise in a cold room. Hand exercise can be done in a basin of warm water.

When Have You Done Too Much?

Listen to the signals your body gives you. A general rule of thumb is that if exercise-induced pain lasts longer than two hours, cut back. Do not stop.

Any exercise programme is bound to have setbacks, but these are not permanent. If you experience exercise-induced pain for longer than two hours, decrease the number of repetitions or be less forceful. If that does not help, choose a different exercise that is more appropriate for you.

Types of Exercises

Depending on your type of arthritis and your overall health, your doctor may prescribe many different exercises for you.

Passive exercises are those in which your doctor or therapist moves your arm, hand, or leg through its normal range of motion and you exert no effort. Active exercises are those that you do with the assistance of a trained person to increase both the range of motion of a joint and the strength of muscles. If you cannot straigthen your knee fully by yourself, for example, you may be able to do so with a little help. Over a period of weeks or even months, improvements may be made. Resistance exercises are those in which you work against some type of pressure or force. For example, you may be asked to push your foot against pressure applied by the hand of another person, or you may use weights. Resistance exercises are particularly good for strengthening weakened muscles.

Your physician and physical therapist will outline your individualized daily exercise plan. But to give you an idea of what your exercises might include, some examples included in a home care manual produced by the US Arthritis Foundation follow. These exercises were designed for individuals who do not have severe joint damage or marked weakness. Before beginning any of these exercise, please consult your physician or physical therapist.

Range-of-Motion Exercises: *Range-of-motion* or stretching exercises mean how far in various directions each joint can be moved by the muscles attached to it. In other words these exercises involve moving a joint as far as it will comfortably go through its full range of motion or stretch. To prevent loss of motion and deformity and to minimize stiffness, you should move each joint through its complete range of motion everyday.

Range-of-motion exercises help maintain normal joint movement or restore movement if it has been lost.

Learn how far your joints can and should be able to move normally. To make sure you get full motion, move your joint to the point of pain, hold it there for a moment, and then move a little bit farther. If a joint is inflamed and painful, however, be gentle as you move through your motions. Perform as many of them as you can by yourself; sometimes you may need a helper, and when you do, your helper should not use force. Exercises on pages 79 to 90 illustrate range-of-motion exercises for various joints.

Strengthening Exercises: Strengthening exercises help maintain or increase the strength and power of your muscles. Two kinds of strengthening exercises are commonly recommended for arthritis patients: resistive and isometric. In resistive exercises the joint is actively exercised against resistance, such as a weight. These exercises are usually prescribed individually and are not shown here. However, if you are advised to do resistive exercises, be sure that you understand the specific amount of weight you should use and how many times you should repeat each exercise each day.

In isometric exercises you strongly tighten the muscle but do not move the joint. Isometric exercises are generally a safe and effective way to increase your strength and can be particularly helpful for individuals with painful joints because the muscle can be strengthened with a minimum amount of joint motion. Also, these exercises can be done at almost any time or place because the only movement necesssary is tightening and relaxing the muscles. Usually the tightened muscle is held fo a slow count of five. Then you relax, rest a minute, and repeat the exercise. Exercises on pages 90 to 94 illustrate examples of these exercises.

Positioning Exercises: When started early in the course of arthritis, these exercises can help prevent deformity. In rheumatoid arthritis the shoulders, hands, hips, and knees are particularly susceptible to stiffness and deformity. By regularly placing your body in certain positions, you can help prevent predictable deformity in these joints.

You can use these positions as self-tests to make sure you are maintaining the normal range of motion for your joints and to keep track of your progress in your exercise programme. If you find any exercises difficult or unusually painful, consult your physician or physical therapist.

Exercises on pages 95 and 96 illustrate some examples of positioning exercises.

Limbering Up Exercises: You can help reduce morning stiffness or stiffness after staying in one position too long by doing the range-of-motion exercises each day only a few times to loosen up.

Even before you get out of bed you can do two or three repetitions of the soulder, wrist, knee and hip exercises. At times you might want to take a warm shower or bath first and then lie down on the bed again to do the exercises. Either way, it is important to get your body moving comfortably as soon as possible.

You can also do the limbering up routine during the day whenever your joints feel stiff.

Following your exercise programme every day is an important part of your total treatment programme that should enable you to manage your arthritis well and maintain the best possible function and independence, advises the US Arthritis Foundation.

RANGE-OF-MOTION OR STRETCHING EXERCISES

Joint Involved: Shoulder

Exercise 1*: Lie on your back. Raise one arm over your head, keeping your elbow straight. Try to bring your arm close to your ear. Return your arm slowly to your side. Repeat this exercise with your other arm. Repeat, alternating arms.

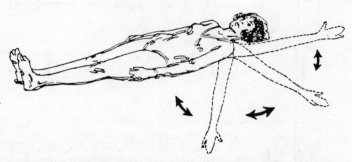

Exercise 2*: Clasp your hands behind your back. Move your hands up your back to midback. Return down to buttocks and repeat. Remember to keep your head and back erect.

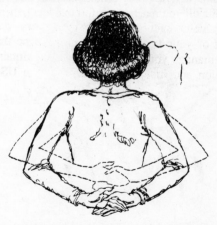

---

* All exercises marked * are included in this book with permission of the US Arthritis Foundation.

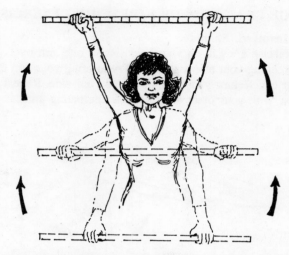

Exercise 3: Stand upright and hold a cane or a stick firmly from both ends with your arms extended fully forward. Raise the cane or stick as high overhead as possible. You might try doing this in front of a mirror. You don't have to move both ends to the same height—play around with it. Try raising it to different heights till you reach a comfortable level, then gradually increase your lift.

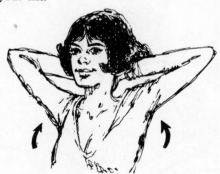

Joints Involved: Shoulder and Elbow
    Exercise 4: Clasp your hands behind your head. Move your elbows back as far as you can. As you move your elbows back, pull your chin in. Return to starting position and repeat.

Exercise 5*: With the forearm resting firmly on a tabletop and the hand hanging over the edge of the table, bend your wrist up as far as possible. Hold. Bend your wrist down as far as possible. Hold. Repeat.

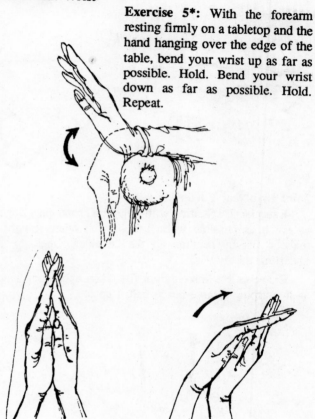

Exercise 6: a) Place your hands together by joining the palms and keeping the fingers straight. b) Press the right hand backward with the left hand, then reverse and press the left hand backward with the right hand. *Exert pressure at the palm* and not on the fingertips. Bend the wrist just as much as possible.

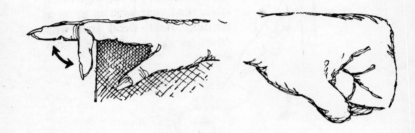

Joint Involved: Fingers

Exercise 7*: Starting with fingertips, bend each finger joint as much as possible while keeping the other straight. Then make a fist by bending all the knuckles. Open the fist by uncurling the fingers.

Exercise 8*: Make a tight fist. Then open your hand wide as if grasping a large beach ball. Repeat.

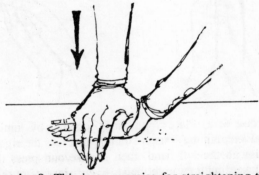

Exercise 9: This is an exercise for straightening the joints of the fingers. Place your hand as flat as possible on a table and then place your other hand across your fingers and gently press down, straightening the fingers.

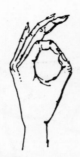
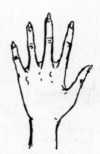

Exercise 10: Try to form a letter "O" with each finger and thumb. a) Touch the tip of the thumb to the tip of the index finger, then b) spread your fingers as wide as possible. Proceed on to touch the tip of the thumb to the tips of your other fingers, spreading the fingers wide after each attempt. If you cannot quite bring the thumb to touch the finger, use the other hand to help them bring together gently.

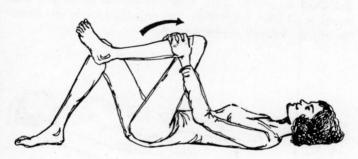

Joint Involved: Knee

Exercise 11: Lie on your back. Bend your knees. Keep your feet flat. Bring your knee towards your chest. Gently bend the knee with your hands and try to touch your heel to your buttock. Do this exercise, one leg at a time.

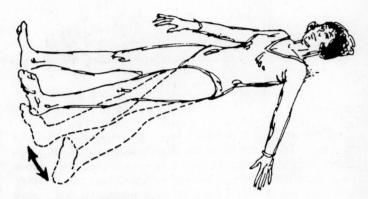

Joint Involved: Hip

Exercise 12*: Lie flat on your back with your legs straight and about six inches apart. Slide one leg out to the side and return, at all times keeping the toes pointing straight up toward the ceiling. Repeat, alternating legs.

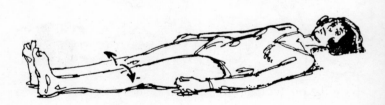

Exeercise 13*: Lie flat on your back with your legs straight and about six inches apart. Roll your knees out, keeping your knees straight, Repeat.

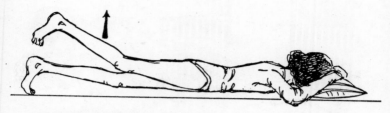

Exercise 14: This exercise helps to increase the backward motion of the hip. Lie face down. This alone may provide a good stretch for those who spend a great deal of time sitting or in bed. If this position is comfortable, raise your leg as high as possible. This exercise should *not* be done by people with low back or disc problems.

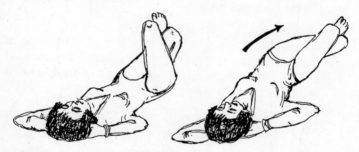

Exercise 15: a) Lie on your back, hands out to the side or behind your head. Bend your hip and knees and place feet flat. Cross your right leg over the left knee. b) Rotate hips to the right, trying to touch the knee to the floor. Keep your upper body flat on the floor. Repeat to the other side.

Benefits: This exercise increases the ability of the hip to rotate (roll in and out). This is important for activities such as dancing or rolling over and getting out of bed. This is also a good exercise for stretching the low and middle back, but some may find it too strenuous for the back.

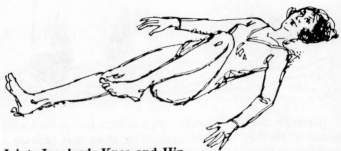

Joints Involved: Knee and Hip

Exercise 16*: Lie on your back. Bend one knee up towards your chest as far as possible. Then return your leg slowly, straightening your knee. Repeat this exercise with your other leg. Repeat, alternating legs.

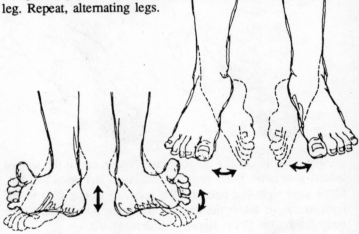

Joint Involved: Ankle

Exercise 17*: Sit in a chair with your feet flat on the floor. Keeping your heels down, lift the rest of your feet up as high as possible. Then, keeping the front of your feet on the floor, lift your heels up as high as possible.

Exercise 18*: Finally, turn the soles of both feet toward each other, then turn them away from each other. Repeat.

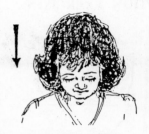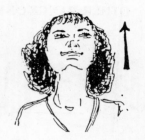

Joint Involved: Neck

Exercise 19: Slowly drop your chin to your chest, then slowly raise your head and very gently drop the head backward. Do not proceed with this exercise if you feel a sharp pain down your arm. Return head to the upright position slowly. *This motion should never be forced.*

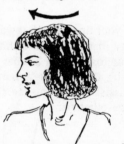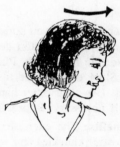

Exercise 20: Turn to look over your right shoulder, then turn to look as far over the left shoulder as possible.

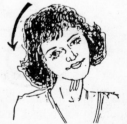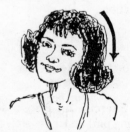

Exercise 21: Tilt your head to the right and then to the left. Try to touch your ear to your shoulder.

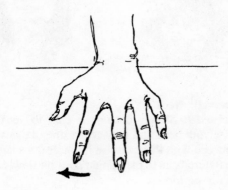

Exercise 22: If you notice that your fingers drift toward the little finger — a common deformity in rheumatoid arthritis — this exercise is for you. Place your forearm on a table, palm down. Slide each finger toward the thumb, not moving the forearm. Use your other hand to assist in pushing the fingers gently if necessary. Repeat with the other hand.

Benefits: The exercise works to keep your knuckles and wrist in correct alignment with your forearm, promoting optimum function.

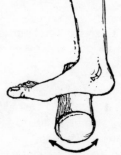

Exercise 23: Place a dowel (large mop handle, closet rod, rolling pin) under the arch of the foot and roll it back and forth.

Benefits: This feels great and it stretches the ligaments of the arch of the foot.

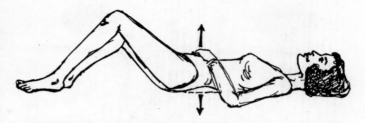

Exercise 24: Lie on the bed or floor with both knees bent, feet flat. Place your hands on your abdomen. Flatten the small of your back against the floor by tightening your buttocks and pulling in your stomach. If this concept is difficult for you, think of bringing your pubic bone toward your chin. Once you have mastered the pelvic tilt in the lying position, try it while standing and sitting.

Benefits: This exercise is good for low back problems.

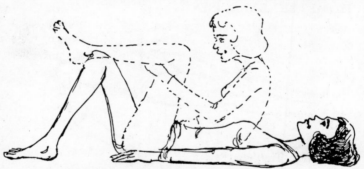

Exercise 25: For a low back stretch, lie on the floor, keeping your knees bent, feet flat. Bring one knee toward your chin, using your hands to assist with the stretch. Maintain this position for five seconds and lower the leg slowly. Repeat with the other knee. To stretch the upper and middle back at the same time, raise your head and shoulder from the floor as you bring your knee toward your chin. *If this creates or increases neck pain, discontinue this portion of the exercise.*

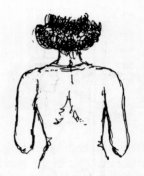 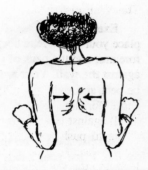

Exercise 26: Sit on the edge of a bed or chair. Squeeze your shoulder blades together by moving your elbows as far back as possible.

Benefits: This is a good exercise for the middle and upper back.

ISOMETRIC EXERCISES

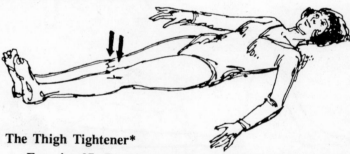

The Thigh Tightener*

Exercise 27: Exercises for the quardriceps muscle in the front of the thigh are valuable in rheumatoid arthritis for preventing bent-knee deformities. Lying flat on your back, attempt to push your right knee down into the bed or floor. You should be tightening the muscle on the front of your thigh. Hold this for a slow count of five. Relax. Repeat with the left leg. Alternate and repeat for each leg five times.

90

The Wallpusher*

Exercise 28: Face a wall and place your elbow, the back of your forearm, and the back of your hand against the wall. Your arms should be bent at a right angle. Push your entire forearm (elbow, wrist and hand) against the wall as if you are trying to push the wall away. Be sure you stand up straight. Do *not* lean into the wall. Hold for a slow count of five. Release. Repeat five times with one arm, then five times with the other arm. You can also do this exercise while sitting in a chair and pushing against the arm of the chair.

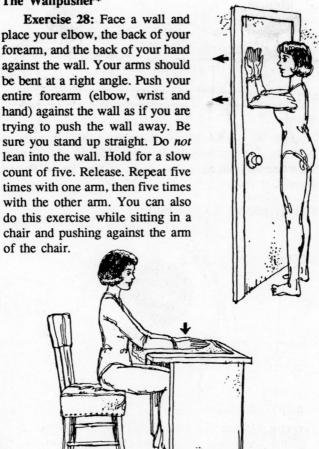

The Deskholder*

Exercise 29: Sit in a chair at a table. Place a towel on the table and rest the front of your forearm and hand down against the towel. Hold for a slow count of five. Relax. Repeat five times with each arm.

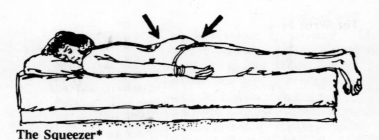

The Squeezer*

Exercise 30: This exercise is for the gluteal muscles in your buttocks. Lie flat on your stomach. Sqeeze your buttock muscles together. Hold for a slow count of five. Relax. Repeat five times.

STRENGTHENING EXERCISES

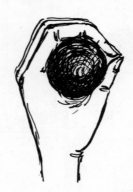

The Finger Press

Exercise 31: This exercise is for strengthening the muscles that bend the fingers to pick up objects. Lightly press the tip of the thumb to the tip of the index finger. Hold for six seconds, maintaining a perfect "O" shape, then relax. Continue lightly pressing the tip of the thumb to the tip of each finger. To help maintain the "O" shape, place a pill bottle or any other cylinder in your hand. Those with rheumatoid arthritis should not press the fingers together but just touch them lightly.

The Wrist Press

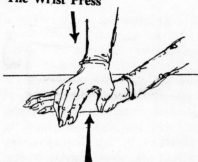

Exercise 32: This exercise is for strengthening the muscles that bend and straighten the wrist. Place your hand on a table or arm rest. Place the heel of the other hand on top. Raise the bottom hand, pushing against the top hand. Hold for six seconds, then relax. Reverse positions of the hand and repeat. Remember, while you are pressing the hands together, allow no joint movement. If it is painful to use your other hand as the stationary object, try to lift the hand against another stable object, such as the chair arm.

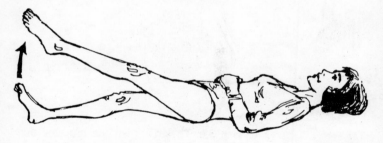

The Straight-Leg Raise

Exercise 33: To strengthen the muscles that bend the hip as well as the muscle that runs across the front of the knee do this exercise. Lie on your back. Keep your arms in a comfortable position. Tighten the muscle that runs across the front of the knee and then raise your leg one to two feet above the ground, keeping the knee straight. Do not arch your back. Hold for six seconds. Relax. If you have low back discomfort you should do this exercise with the other knee bent.

The Tiptoe

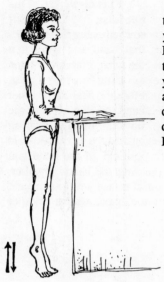

Exercise 34: Lightly hold a table for support. a) Raise up on your tiptoes. Hold for six seconds. Lower slowly. This exercise maybe too stressful for some, especially if you are overweight. b) As an alternative exercise, place the sole of your foot against a stationary object (wall, chair leg) and push. Hold for six seconds and then relax.

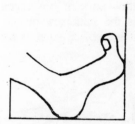

The Back Push

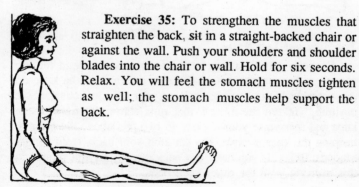

Exercise 35: To strengthen the muscles that straighten the back, sit in a straight-backed chair or against the wall. Push your shoulders and shoulder blades into the chair or wall. Hold for six seconds. Relax. You will feel the stomach muscles tighten as well; the stomach muscles help support the back.

POSITIONING EXERCISES
The Mark*

Exercise 36: Facing a wall or door frame, reach up and mark the highest spot you can touch with your fingertips; this mark becomes your self-test point. Touch the mark once each day. Alternate arms. As long as you can touch the mark you are maintaining your normal range. If you can go higher, mark your new spot. It becomes your new check-point.

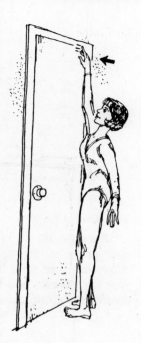

The Motion Test*

Exercise 37: Lying on your stomach with your feet hanging over the edge of the bed is an excellent way to check the motion in your legs. When using this position as a self-test, be sure that both hips are flat on the bed and that both knees are straight. See how far you can move your legs to each side and upward.

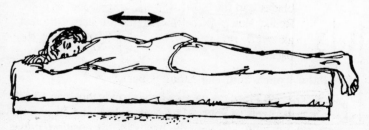

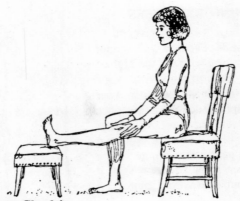

The Knee Check*

Exercise 38: Sit in a chair. Place one foot up on another chair or on an ottoman. This is a good position in which to make sure your knee is not getting stiff. With your foot up, your knee should be straight. Check both knees. If your knee doesn't straighten, consult your physician.

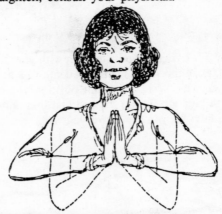

The Palm Touch and The Elbow Check*

Exercise 39: Place the palms of your hands together. Check to see that the heels of your palms, your palms, and all of your fingers are touching, and with the hands in this position, move your elbows straight out to the side without separating your palms. Return. Repeat.

96

Physical Therapy

Exercise and physical therapy may be considered synonymous. Physical therapy is exercise of a specific type. It may be the exercises you are advised to do at home or a routine that your physical therapist does with you at the health centre.

For osteoarthritis, physical therapy is prescribed to help keep the joints flexible, to preserve the strength of muscles on which the joints depend for stability, and to protect diseased joints against further damaging stress. Because osteoarthritis tends to be progressive, physical therapy must be carried on indefinitely. Often physical therapy treatment begins in a hospital or health centre setting and then plans are outlined for patients to do at home, either alone or with the help of another person.

In all types of arthritis the purpose of physical therapy is to help a patient make the best use of remaining abilities and to restore the maximum degree of physical function. With a little effort muscle weakness and loss of normal joint motion can be prevented or corrected.

Components of Your Treatment Plan

Rest, exercise and physical therapy are important components of the treatment plan in arthritis. Sometimes a daily routine of many 10-to-15-minute rest periods helps people who have arthritis. Some plan to rest awhile each day after their at-home exercise sessions. Each individual seems to be able to find the routine that is most convenient and makes him or her most comfortable.

Individuals with rheumatoid arthritis may feel extremely tired at times, and those are the times for additional rest periods and reduction of activities.

All parts of your arthritis treatment plan will interact. In addition to rest and exercise, what you eat is important. Diet in arthritis can help you reduce your weight, which puts extra stress on weight-bearing joints. You will read more about controlling weight and improving your overall health through better nutrition in Chapter 7.

7

What is a Good Diet for Arthritis?

Can a good diet be especially helpful in arthritis? The answer is both yes and no. No special foods or diets can cure arthritis or make it go away. However, by helping you deal with other related problems (such as over-weight) and helping you feel more fit and energetic proper nutrition can help you cope better with arthritis.

Over the years many books and articles have been published proclaming a wide variety of special diets and food supplements and vitamins as arthritis *cures*. If you or someone close to you has arthritis, you have undoubtedly read or heard about some of these claims.

Responsible scientists have made many careful studies designed to find out whether there is any link between diet and arthritis. These medical experts have found little scientific evidence that any food or diet causes arthritis or that any special diet or food or vitamin can cure it. Gout is an exception. It is the only form of arthritis in which diet may be a factor.

In all forms of arthritis, the most helpful diet is a normal diet that is nourishing and well balanced. Good nutrition is important to good health for everyone. For someone who has arthritis, good meals and nutritious food are even more important to help the body cope with the stresses of this long-term disease.

Your physician and health team will help you with personal diet concerns such as maintaining proper weight and making adjustments in your diet to counteract the possible side effects of some medications.

You can help yourself a great deal if you eat a varied, nourishing diet. On the following pages are some suggestions that may make it easier for you to plan a good diet you need.

The Basic Four Food Groups

The simplest way to make sure you eat a balanced diet is to eat some foods every day from each of the basic four food groups. These four are meat and other proteins; milk and milk products; fruits and vegetables; and breads and cereal foods.

The meat group includes poultry, fish, eggs, cheese, beans and peas, nuts, seeds, and peanut butter. These foods provide protein (as do milk products and many vegetables), which is essential for maintenance and repair of body tissues. They also supply iron for red blood cells, other minerals, vitamins, and some fat. Adults, teenagers, and children should have two servings a day of foods from this group.

Milk and milk products, including yoghurt, cheese, and ice cream, are important as a source of calcium to maintain bones and teeth and to keep the nervous system healthy. Milk products also provide protein, some vitamins and fat. Adults need two servings a day; teenagers need four; children need two or three. A serving is 240 gms of milk or yoghurt, 1-1/2 cups of ice cream, or a little more than 30 gms of hard cheese.

Vegetables and fruits provide important vitamins and minerals. They also supply us with dietary fibre to help keep the digestive system operating smoothly. Everyone should have four servings a day. A serving is one potato or apple or a half cup of chopped vegetables or fruits.

One serving from this group every day should be rich in vitamin C—orange or tomato juice, for instance, or strawberries or cantaloupe.

One serving, at least every other day, should be high in

vitamin A — one of the deep green or yellow vegetables and fruits, including carrots, sweet potatoes, broccoli, greens, apricots, and peaches.

The whole grain and enriched breads, cereals, and pasta foods provide carbohydrates for food energy. They also supply some protein, minerals and vitamins, and dietary fibre. Everyone should have at least four servings a day. A serving is one slice of bread, half a cup of pasta or rice, or a bowl of cereal.

In addition to foods from these groups, the diet should include some butter, salad oil, or other fat, for fat-soluble vitamins and essential fatty acids. Some simple desserts, such as puddings, may be added if you need extra calories.

Variety in Your Diet

One other important rule for good nutrition is to eat a wide variety of foods. More than 40 different vitamins, minerals, and other nutrients are essential to health and are available to your body only from the food you eat. No single food has all the nutrients you need. Egg, for example, is almost a perfect package of nutrition, but has no vitamin C. Milk, which is designed as the sole nourishment for infants or animals, contains no iron.

By eating as many different foods as possible, you are likely to get all the nutrients you need. You will also get foods with a variety of tastes and textures, and that will make your meals more interesting.

There is another reason for eating a variety of foods. Some people who have chronic diseases like arthritis believe that after they eat a particular food, their condition changes for the worse. If that happens, it's only sensible to stop eating the food that is believed to cause the problem. If you are eating a varied diet, the nutrients you lose from one food will easily by replaced by the same nutrients from other foods.

You're also likely to get better nutritional value when you use more fresh fruits and vegetables and meats and foods that have had only a miminim of processing. Frankfurters and cold cuts, for instance, have less protein and more fat than the same amount of lean meat. Whole grain bread has all the original nutrients from the grain. Enriched bread has a number of nutrients removed when the flour is milled; enrichment replaces some of them, but not all.

Controlling Your Weight

A good diet should help you stay at your normal weight.

To find out what is a good weight for you, look at a height and weight table that shows ideal weights. Ten percent more or less than the ideal weight is considered to be within the normal range.

If your weight is normal, and you are not gaining or losing any, your diet is giving you enough energy from food, measured in calories, to balance the food energy, or calories, you burn up in the activities of daily living. To estimate how many calories you should be getting in your daily diet, multiply your ideal weight by 30. If your ideal weight, for instance, is 65 kg, your diet should give you a total of 1,950 calories a day. If you want to find out how many calories you are actually getting, write down all the foods you eat during a day, including the amounts, and check the calorie count in the calorie table you can find in most diet books.

Underweight

With arthritis you may sometimes find that you are not very hungry, you are eating less and losing weight, you are feeling tired and run-down, and you have less resistance to colds and other infections. At these times you may need extra nourishment and more high-calorie foods in your diet.

If you think you are underweight, ask your physician for a plan that will help you gain weight.

If your appetite is poor, snacking between meals may help you increase your overall calorie intake. Half a sandwich, milk and a cookie, or cheese and crackers would all be good choices. Time the snacks so you'll be hungry again at mealtime. Eating with someone else for company may also help you eat better.

Having company at mealtime makes it a pleasant occasion, and this is likely to improve your appetite. If you live alone, share a meal occasionally with a neighbour or a friend. Each of you can prepare part of the meal, so no one feels burdened. Or have your meal on tray in front of the TV set with your local channel programme for company.

Overweight

Overweight is also a problem for many people who have arthritis. Some tend to put on kilograms because they are not physically active. The excess weight places an added burden on weight-bearing joints and contributes to increased pain and inflammation.

If this happens, your physician or nutritionist can give you suggestions for an appropriate weight-loss diet. The techniques described below may make it easier to follow a diet, take weight off and keep it off.

Hints for Losing Weight

Cut down fat in your daily diet. Fat has more than twice as many calories as protein and carbohydrates (9 to the gram, compared to 4). Trim visible fat from meat, remove the skin from poultry, use low-fat milk, and cut back on fatty foods like butter, oil-based salad dressings, and gravies.

Cut down on refined sugar, rich sweets and desserts, and alcoholic drinks. They give you a lot of calories but few or none of the vitamins and other nutrients your body needs.

Eat more slowly. It takes bout 20 minutes for the appetite control centre in the brain to let you know you've had enough and aren't hungry anymore. It will help you slow down if you put down your knife and fork between bites, have a drink of water, or stop to talk to others at the table.

Don't eat because you're tired or bored. If you're tired, take a nap or rest in a comfortable chair. If it's nervous tension, physical activity is better than food. Wash dishes, pull up weeds or go for a walk if you can. If you're bored, instead of eating, read a book, phone a friend, or straighten your bureau drawers.

Ideal Weight for Men over 25 years

Height			Weight	
Feet	Inches	Cm.	Lbs	Kg.
5	2	157.5	118 — 129	53.5 — 58.5
5	3	160.0	121 — 133	54.9 — 60.3
5	4	162.6	124 — 136	56.2 — 61.7
5	5	165.1	127 — 139	57.6 — 63.0
5	6	167.6	130 — 143	59.0 — 64.9
5	7	170.2	134 — 147	60.8 — 66.7
5	8	172.7	138 — 152	62.6 — 68.9
5	9	175.3	142 — 156	64.4 — 70.8
5	10	177.8	146 — 160	66.2 — 72.6
5	11	180.3	150 — 165	68.0 — 74.8
6	0	182.9	154 — 170	69.9 — 77.1
6	1	185.4	158 — 175	71.7 — 79.4
6	2	188.0	162 — 180	73.5 — 81.6

Ideal Weight for Women over 25 years

Height			Weight	
Feet	Inches	Cm.	Lbs	Kg.
4	10	147.3	96 — 107	43.5 — 48.5
4	11	149.9	98 — 110	44.5 — 49.9
5	0	152.4	101 — 113	45.8 — 51.3
5	1	154.9	104 — 116	47.2 — 52.6
5	2	157.5	107 — 119	48.5 — 54.0
5	3	160.0	110 — 122	49.9 — 55.3
5	4	162.6	113 — 126	51.3 — 57.2
5	5	165.1	116 — 130	52.6 — 59.0
5	6	167.6	120 — 135	54.4 — 61.2
5	7	170.2	124 — 139	56.2 — 63.0
5	8	172.7	128 — 143	58.1 — 64.9
5	9	175.3	132 — 147	59.9 — 66.7
5	10	177.8	136 — 151	61.7 — 68.5
5	11	180.3	140 — 155	63.5 —70.3
6	0	182.9	144 — 159	65.3 — 72.0

Diet and Gout

Gout is one form of arthritis in which food may be a factor. Gout is caused by uric acid crystals deposited in and around the joints.

To help prevent painful attacks of gout, many physicians recommend that their patients avoid foods that increase the body's production of uric acid. Such foods include liver and other organ meats, anchovies, sardines, peas and beans. Because heavy consumption of alcohol can also bring on a gout attack, abstinence is a sensible idea.

In recent years, however, because of effective medications, the role of diet in gout is becoming less a factor, and many people with gout take their medication while not giving up any of their favourite foods.

Gout patients, like others with arthritis, should watch their weight because excess weight increases the stress on painful joints. The physician or nutritionist can suggest a weight-loss programme. Fasting to lose weight is not advisable; it has been known to lead to a gout attack, since fasting has been associated with an elevation of the serum uric acid.

Helping Yourself

What you eat is largely your decision. If you shop and cook for yourself, or if you plan the shopping and cooking and it is done by others, your food preferences can be followed closely. While improving your general nutrition is one of the many factors that interrelate to improve your health, your diet may be the one factor over which you have most control. Help yourself to health by following the diet plan recommended to you by your health care team and learning all you can about good nutrition.

8

Making Each Day Easier

Look at how you live — what kinds of activities you do, which ones are the most important, and how you perform them. There may be easier ways to do many of them.

Your physician and physical or occupational therapist will counsel you on a variety of activities that might include how to cook, how to get on and off a bus, how to relax and relieve tension, and how to continue to enjoy a happy love life. In this chapter you will find reminders for some of the hints you may already have heard and perhaps some additional helpful ideas. A wide variety of aids for individuals with arthritis is available. Sources are listed in Chapter 12.

Daily Objectives

It's rarely easy to change habits, but at this time, it may be helpful to make some changes to avoid discomfort, save energy, and protect your joints.

Avoid Activities That Cause Prolonged Pain

You will be able to detect the difference between pain and discomfort. Avoid letting pain last longer than 15 to 20 minutes. Performing exercises may make you uncomfortable if you haven't done them for a while, just as it does in individuals who don't have arthritis. Keep this in mind when you do housework, participate in sports, or do the exercises outlined in Chapter 6.

Save Energy

Look at your day-to-day and week-to-week activities carefully. Make a schedule that includes your social and leisure activities as well as your work and chores.

Try to spread your difficult and stressful tasks throughout the week. For example, if you try to do all your shopping and errands in one day, you may find that walking is exhausting and painful, whereas you could better tolerate several short trips during the week. Don't start complicated activities that you can't stop, if they make you feel uncomfortable.

It is important for you to plan and take rest periods, whether you have a job or stay at home. The best position is one in which your muscles and joints are at rest. If possible, lie down. If you have been standing, get off your feet. If you have been sitting, get up and move around. Frequent breaks from your routine will often allow you extra energy to enjoy social activities at the end of the day.

Joint Protection

You can protect your joints by changing positions frequently to prevent stiffness, taking care to avoid joint positions that may be painful, or placing excessive pressure or stress on joints, as in kneeling and heavy lifting. Slide heavy objects where possible to avoid putting stress on your hands. Sit when possible, preventing excess stress on lower extremities. For example, use a stool in the kitchen when preparing meals, doing dishes, or ironing. Have chairs and desks at home and at work at correct heights, preventing strain on your back. Avoid low chairs, which stress the knees, when getting up or sitting down.

CARING FOR YOUR JOINTS

Simple everyday tasks involve almost all body joints. We can care and look after our joints by performing these tasks in a correct way; or we can cause undue stress on our joints and perhaps even damage them. In the following pages, the right and the wrong ways of performing everyday tasks are illustrated.

Pushing Up From A Chair

Avoid using your writs or knuckles when getting up from a chair.

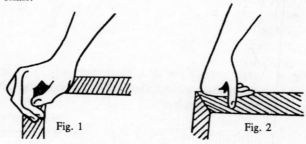

Fig. 1   Fig. 2

Avoid these methods. They cause pain. The knuckles come under extreme stress (as in Fig. 2).

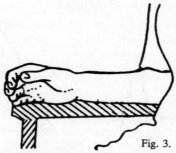

Fig. 3.

Use your forearm(s) to push or get up from a chair; it distributes the weight more evenly.

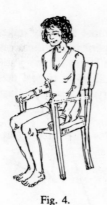
Fig. 4.

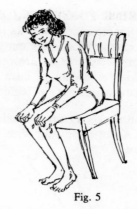
Fig. 5

Fig. 4: When getting out of a chair, one way is to lean forward with your hands around your knees and push up/stand up by using your leg muscles.

Fig. 5: Another way of getting up from a chair is to distribute the weight between your forearms and the legs. This avoids straining the knuckles or the shoulders.

Carrying A Bag
Avoid carrying too much weight.

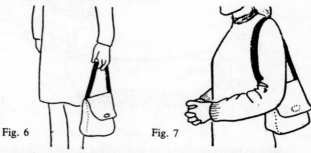
Fig. 6   Fig. 7

Fig. 6: You may strain your shoulders and fingers if you carry your bag by holding the strap.

Fig. 7: Carry your bag on your shoulder if it is not too heavy.

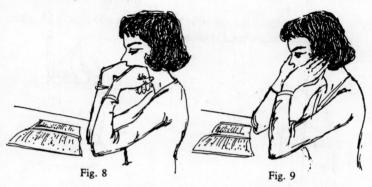

Fig. 8   Fig. 9

Fig. 8: Avoid resting your face on your elbows and knuckles when reading a book.

Fig. 9: Avoid resting your face on your elbows and wrists when reading a book.

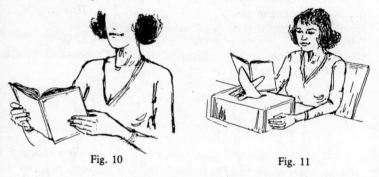

Fig. 10   Fig. 11

Fig. 10: Avoid holding the book too tightly. It can strain the wrist.

Fig. 11: Use a bookrest. It avoids any strain on your elbows, knuckles, wrists and neck.

Opening A Jar

Avoid holding the lid with your fingers and thumb to open a jar. It can strain your thumb.

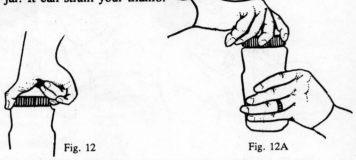

Fig. 12

Fig. 12A

Figs. 12 & 12A: The entire load is on the fingers and thumb.

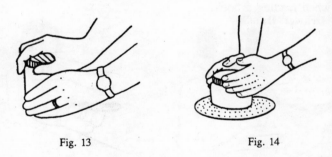

Fig. 13

Fig. 14

Fig. 13: To increase your grip on the jar use both hands. Use the palm of the hand to increase the grip and always screw open towards the thumb.

Fig. 14: Both hands can also be used to hold the lid after keeping the jar on a non-slip mat or damp cloth.

Opening Tins

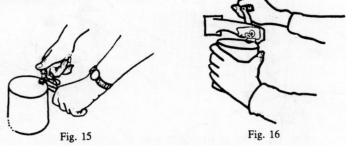

Fig. 15   Fig. 16

Fig. 15: Avoid using a hand tin-opener when opening tins. It puts strain on the wrist.

Fig. 16: Use a wall-mounted tin-opener with a shelf underneath to hold the weight of the container.

Drawer Handles

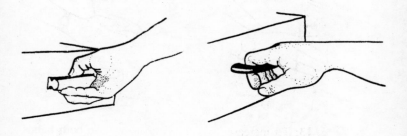

Fig. 17   Fig. 18

Fig. 17: Avoid having drawer handles which have to be held between the thumb and the fingers for pulling the drawer out. These may strain all the finger joints.

Fig. 18: Use drawer handles as shown here. These handles distribute the weight more evenly without straining the fingers.

Using A Teapot
A lightweight or half-filled teapots will help.

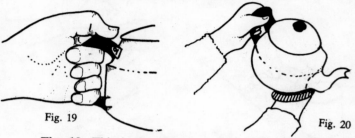

Fig. 19   Fig. 20

Fig. 19: This is the right way to hold the handle. Use a teapot with larger handle.

Fig. 20: Use both hands to hold the teapot. This distributes the weight on the wrist and forearm.

Holding A Cup

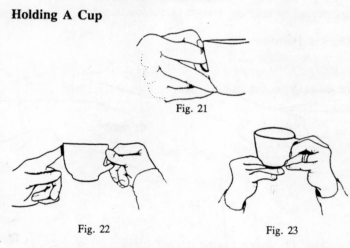

Fig. 21

Fig. 22   Fig. 23

Fig. 21: Avoid holding a cup this way. It causes strain on fingers and knuckles.

Figs. 22 & 23: Use both hands to hold a lightweight cup or a mug. Cups with larger handles help.

Carrying Dishes

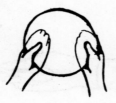 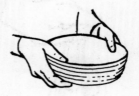

Fig. 24.

Fig. 24: Avoid carrying dishes in one hand. It causes strain on the wrist and thumb. Use both hands. Even with both hands there is still wrist strain; but it is a workable compromise.

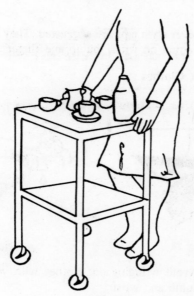

Fig. 25.

Fig. 25: If you can, avoid carrying dishes even on a tray. It can cause strain on your neck, shoulders, elbows, wrist and fingers. It is best to use a trolley.

Taps

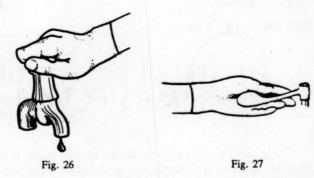

Fig. 26   Fig. 27

Fig. 26: Most bib type taps cause strain on wrist, thumb and fingers.

Fig. 27: Lever style taps are suggested. They minimise the effort and the strain on wrist, thumb and fingers.

Wringing Out Clothes

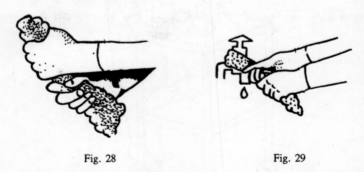

Fig. 28   Fig. 29

Fig. 28: Avoid wringing out clothes with your hands. It strains your thumb and wrist.

Fig. 29: For a workable compromise twist the clothes around a tap and use both hands to twist and wring.

Relieving Back Strain

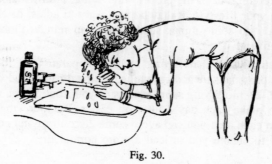

Fig. 30.

Fig. 30: Avoid bending like this over a basin. It you are washing hair, use a hand shower.

Relieving Back Strain

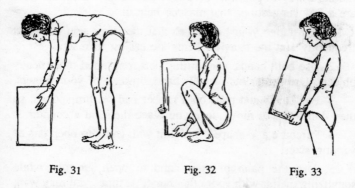

Fig. 31   Fig. 32   Fig. 33

Fig. 31: Avoid lifting a load/weight this way. It can strain your back.

Figs. 32 & 33: This is a right way. Bend your knees, rest your weight equally on both feet, hold the load close to your body and lift.

Activities of Daily Life

It is important to be active and maintain good movement and strength, but in the proper way. While arthritis should not dictate your lifestyle, it may be necessary to adjust or alter the way you do some things so that you can remain mobile and independent.

Activities of daily living include preparation of food and eating, personal care and grooming, getting dressed, and walking around. By modifying some aspects of your routine you may be able to make each day a little bit easier. By following a few hints in each area you can avoid some discomfort and conserve energy to enable you to lead a more normal life.

Preparing Food and Eating

Good nutrition is essential to your good health. If you prepare your own food, you must be able to perform a variety of kitchen chores. And if you are responsible for preparing your family's meals, you will want to continue your routine in as normal a way as possible, even though you have arthritis. Here are a few suggestions that may be helpful:

1. Rearrange your kitchen so that the items you use most frequently and the heaviest items are easiest to reach.

2. Use both hands when lifting pots, pans, and other heavy objects. Use the palms of your hands instead of your fingers.

3. Put bowls and pans on a rubber pad or thin sponge, so they don't slip or move once you place them on a counter.

4. Purchase a V-shaped wall unit with teeth, to open jars of varying sizes.

5. Use the palm of your hand to open jar tops while stabilizing the jar with your other hand. At times you may want to ask the person at the check-out counter at your supermarket to loosen the top of a jar for you.

6. Use an electric can opener instead of a manual one.

7. A pegboard will enable you to organize kitchen items inexpensively and efficiently within your reach. Use hangers

with prongs for the pegboard, so that they stay in place. Brackets for shelves and various holders can keep your various kitchen tools handy and orderly.

8. Drawer dividers may enable you to pick up one item without moving others. With kitchen implements arranged this way you can use tongs, instead of your fingers, to pick up utensils.

9. Make use of lazy Susans or revolving food stand or containers as much as possible in cabinets and on counters. They eliminate the need to grasp many small items repeatedly.

10. Plan your week's menu ahead of time. Cook double or triple portions at one time to reduce preparation and cleanup time. Refrigerate or freeze extra servings.

11. Vary your menu with one-dish meals, which you can find in many cook books.

12. Select appliances carefully to meet your needs. For example, a blender or food processor will reduce stress on your hands.

13. When cutting, select tools that are well made for most efficient use. Choose large handles that feel comfortable in your hand. Keep the blades sharp, clean them carefully after each use, and store them safely. Work at a comfortable height, with the items being cut on a well-secured board.

14. For kitchen clean-up chores, plan your dishwashing area so that you can sit to work. Organize your space so that your activity flows from one side to the other. If the bottom of your sink is low, it can be raised with a wooden sink rack built of narrow slats. If holding a sponge is difficult, use a sponge mitt.

15. Keep a chair or a high stool in your kitchen for chores that you can do sitting.

16. Use a small wheeled cart to move things back and forth in your house or to the yard instead of carrying objects and making many trips.

17. Learn to use your joints in a protected position. For example, when using a sponge or washing dishes, keep your

fingers extended. When opening a milk carton, use the heels of your hands instead of your thumbs to push back the flanges. Avoid placing too much stress on unstable joints, such as the thumbs. You may also want to avoid putting stress on your thumbs by opening a milk carton with a knife. Divide work between both hands and eliminate finger stress as much as possible.

18. Eating utensils can have handles built up by sponge or foam rubber.

19. Mugs with large handles will allow all of your fingers to assist in holding the cup.

20. Eating soup and other non-solid foods requires rotation of your forearm to keep the utensil level. Swivel spoons are available to help you if you lack that ability.

Personal Care

Personal grooming is important because you will fell better when you know that you look better. In the bathroom safety is an important factor. There are many ways to make your personal routine safer and more efficient. Some of them are listed below:

1. You can purchase a raised toilet seat that will permit you to sit down more easily. It may be as many as six inches higher than the standard seat. Many models are available to fit different toilets. Arm rests can also be purchased to fit around the toilet to give you more stability as you sit down and stand up.

2. Use a non-slip mat in the bathtub.

3. You can purchase various types of grab bars for your bathtub. Check to see if there is a place to install them securely.

4. Use a small stool or chair in the tub to sit to shower or a bath bench that reaches from one side of the tub to the other.

5. Long-handled sponges and brushes are available or can be made, to assist you in washing areas that you can't reach.

6. For those who must use wheelchairs, either routinely or occasionally, it is very important to be sure that the bathroom door is wide enough to accommodate the chair. When purchasing

a wheelchair or when moving, be sure to check these measurement in advance.

Getting Dressed

Many specially designed clothing items are now available for those who require garments that are easier to put on and take off.

1. If you have shoulder or hand problems, it is important to purchase clothes that are loose and open in the front. Velcro fasteners are often used instead of buttons or zippers. Also, special button-hooks and zipper pulls with long handles are available.

2. For women, a variety of bras are available with front closings. For men, clip-on ties are available in all styles.

3. Putting on shoes is difficult for many people with arthritis, especially when hip, knee, or back mobility is somewhat restricted. Your local shoe store or variety store may have a long-handled shoe horn and elastic shoelaces, which you may find helpful. Shoes are also available with Velcro fasterers.

4. Metal tongs can be used to help pull up pants or to reach to the floor or a low drawer to pick up personal items.

Walking Around

Making life easier as you walk around indoors as well as outside is important. You will be able to enjoy more activities when they require less physical effort and produce less stress on painful joints.

1. Wear shoes that fit well and are not too heavy.

2. Avoid sitting in low chairs or sit on a pillow to raise you higher. Try to sit in chairs with armrests. When you get up from the chair, push yourself up from the armrests instead of letting your back muscles do all the work. Move forward to the edge of the chair with your feet on the floor back underneath you. Lean forward and push on the arms of the chair with the palms of your hands. It may help to rock forward several times.

3. Don't plop when sitting down.

4. Avoid climbing stairs whenever possible. Climbing stairs puts much more stress on your knees than walking. When taking stairs, use a railing.

5. When going up stairs, go up with your good leg first and take one step at a time. When descending, put the bad leg down first.

6. When climbing on or off a bus, use the handrail. Ask the driver to pull the bus as close to the curb as possible.

7. When getting in and out of a car, it is generally easier to get into the back seat (of a four-door car). Back into the seat and sit down. Then lift and swing in your legs, using your arms to assist them.

8. For those who are confined to a wheelchair a ramp can be built over the steps to allow access to the outdoors.

9. At times assistance devices such as canes and walkers may be necessary to take the stress off a particular joint. Use of such devices should be discussed with and prescribed by your physician or physical therapist. They must be the correct height and you should be carefully instructed in using them.

10. When using a cane, remember that you use it on the opposite side of your problem area. For example, if your right knee is painful, you will use the cane in your left hand.

Aids and Appliances

Joint pain, due to arthritis, can also be relieved or treated by unloading the joint. Weight reduction (one kilogram weight loss can produce a 3 to 4 kg decrease in load across the joint) is one approach. Using a forearm or axillary crutch on the opposite side will reduce by more than one-half the amount of weight borne by the limb in question. A cane, however, while good for balance, is not as effective in unloading a limb as a crutch. Because the problem in arthritis is likely to be chronic, a fairly permanent and comfortable solution needs to be found. For the patient with rheumatoid arthritis (RA), it is critical that the grip is suited to the deformity in the hand. Platform crutches or platform walker can be used.

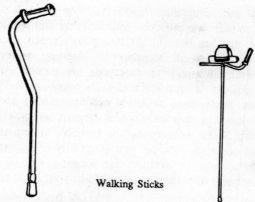

Walking Sticks

Recreation or Leisure Time

Just because you are arthritic does not mean that you have to give up all the sports, recreation and hobbies that you have enjoyed for years. Always remember that your being arthritic need not stop you from taking part in physical activities.

The best form of physical activity is swimming, since the buoyancy of the water helps to support the joints. In addition, much of your normal exercise routine can be performed while in the water.

An embroidery frame that can be attached to a table or chair will allow you to do needle work and sewing without using your hands to stabilize the article.

If you like to play cards, try using a card holder – either you can buy them or easily have them made by sawing a slit in a piece of wood.

When gardening, try sitting on a small stool instead of kneeling to weed and plant.

Health Professionals Can Help You

In addition to your doctor, who will continue to make suggestions to make your daily life easier while you progress with your treatment, other trained health professionals may be helpful. Probably the most important individuals will be the physical and occupational therapists. The physical therapist is trained to help you preserve your mobility and regain physical function that has been lost. Often your physical therapist and physician will work together in planning your treatment programme. Occupational therapists are trained to help you regain skills or learn additional skills necessary for your daily activities. While these skills are productive, they also exercise many joints and muscles, such as fingers, wrists, elbows, and shoulders. Social workers may be available to help you resolve personal concerns, counsel you on family or marital matters, and advise you of avenues for locating various forms of assistance and of resources available in your local community.

Your physician may refer you to one health professional or several who can help you. You will want to become acquainted with them early in the course of your treatment and let them know about your lifestyle so that they may provide assistance to you in as many ways as possible.

Relax More: Reduce Stress

You can't avoid stress completely, but you can reduce it. For example, if noise bothers you when your are uncomfortable, relax in a room away from other family members. Close the door. Play soft music. Use headphones on a stereo set if the kind of music you like isn't the favourite of other family members.

Plan some time each day just for yourself. That may involve taking a walk, reading something unrelated to your job that you enjoy, or watching a favourite program on television. It may mean going to a health club or gym or swimming. Don't wait for free time to do the things you enjoy. Build that free time into each day, and you will feel more relaxed during the remainder of the day.

Don't overplan family or social activities. Try not to be rushed. You may find that just getting ready for an activity takes longer than it once did. Avoid the stress induced by being late. Plan ahead. Allow anough time for necessary preparations. For example, some women with arthritis know that getting ready for a party takes longer because of closing clasps on jewellery and perhaps fastening small buttons. If you have trouble doing certain chores with your fingers, allow extra preparation time to enable you to appear smiling and ready at the appointed time.

Having a chronic disease such as arthritis produces stress for you as well as other members of your family. With chronic discomfort you may find that your temperament is not as even as it once was. At times you may become more irritable with those you love or with whom you work. To compensate for this, think before you react or act. Take sufficient time in making decisions. Keep lines of communication open between yourself and your family members and co-workers. Their understanding of your disease may enable them to keep a calmer attitude about everyday problems. While they shouldn't pamper you, it may be helpful if they can resolve some conflicts without involving you.

Travel as Relaxation

Many people with arthritis find that relaxing away from home for a short time is helpful. Some travel to warmer climates during cold winter months. Others travel to visit friends or relatives in whose company they can rest and enjoy a change of pace.

If you want to travel, discuss your plans with your physician. Generally, anyone who can move around his or her own neighbourhood without assistance can travel with confidence. Advance planning is important, however, if you have any kind of physical disability.

Plane Travel

If you are travelling by air, discuss your limitations with the airline reservations clerk or your travel agent. Airlines offer many special services for persons with limited mobility, such as early boarding, advance seat selection, wheelchairs, and speical meals. The following suggestions may be helpful:

1. Avoid rush days and hours.
2. Take day flights whenever possible. Traveling at night

can be tiresome and cut into your sleeping time.

3. Allow additional time to make connecting flights.

4. Book non-stop flights or direct flights whenever possible, so you do not have to change planes.

5. Ask questions and give airline personnel opportunity to make helpful suggestions to make your trip more pleasant.

6. If you travel with your own wheelchair, ask about regulations regarding its transportation.

Cruises

Many cruises offer accessibility to persons with limited mobility. Some have built-in ramps and extra-wide doorways, specially designed staterooms for handicapped passengers, and other rooms that can be adapted temporarily. If you are interested in a cruise, the following tips may be helpful:

1. Consider the ease of getting to the point of origin of the cruise.

2. Find out if the ship will dock or anchor off shore and how you will transfer from the ship to a launch to get ashore at various ports.

3. If you use a wheelchair, check with the cruise operator to be sure that your chair meets specifications.

4. If you haven't sailed before, take a short cruise before signing on for a long one.

Trains

Some train stations now have more barrier-free arrangements, making train travel easier for disabled persons. Accessibility to cars and stations varies widely throughout world, so check with the train line or your travel agent to be sure that you will be able to manoeuvre in the stations you must pass through during your trip.

If you plan to travel by train, consider the following questions:

1. Can you move from the street, through the station, to the

train platform, and onto the train?

2. Will someone be available to help you at the station?

3. Can you manage alone or should you travel with a companion?

4. Are the train aisles wide enough for a wheelchair?

5. Can meals be brought to your seat or room if you have difficulty walking through a moving train?

Also, if you have particular disabilities, discuss them with railway personnel when making your travel arrangements. You will find that your trip can be made much more comfortable when you follow specific suggestions made by the railway staff.

Bus Travel

Travelling by bus is possible even if you are in a wheelchair. If you call ahead, a terminal employee can arrange to assist you to the bus. Get complete details about departure and arrival time and arrive early enough to avoid the last-minute crowd boarding the bus. Also note these tips.

1. Weekday travel may be easier than travel on busy weekends.

2. Ask about rest stops. Determine how convenient getting to the restroom at the rear of the bus will be.

3. Find out when and where you may have to change buses.

4. Carry a light snack and beverage with you, in case getting to the terminal restaurant is not convenient for you.

5. Carry an inflatable pillow with you for naps.

Hotel Reservations

When making hotel or motel reservations, ask about ground floor rooms, room-side parking, extrawide doorways, and other features that will make you more comfortable while away from home.

Special Tours

From time to time tour operators schedule tours for handicaped persons. You can obtain information on such tours from your travel agent. Before booking any tour, determine the reliability of the tour operator. Check to see if the organization is a member of a recognized tour operators body. To be a member, tour promoters and agents must conform to certain guidelines.

Generally, it may be easier for you to make your arrangements through a travel agent, who will ask questions about your special needs and make plans for your trip according to those needs. When you have confidence in your travel agent you can relax about the arrangements and enjoy your trip.

Learning Relaxation Techniques

Some people find that learned relaxation techniques can help them live more comfortably with arthritis. For example, some people have learned the technique known as *biofeedback,* which enables them to better understand when they are tense and how to relax certain muscles through mental power. In some biofeedback learning centres, electronic sensors are placed on the body to measure various functions, including blood pressure, heart rate, and skin temperature. The individual, aware of these rates because of an audible sound, learns to control them at will. If you are interested in learning about these techniques, talk with your doctor or physical therapist, who will be able to tell you if the techniques could help you. If you do learn biofeedback techniques, it is important that you get instruction from a qualified instructor at a well-established learning centre.

Technique for Progressive Relaxation of Each Muscle Group

First, for each muscle group of the arms and shoulders :

1. Tense (contract) the muscles, holding until the tension is located (two to five seconds).

2. Feel the tension, notice it carefully. Now release, let the tension slide away, all the way.

3. Feel the difference.

4. Notice the pleasant warmth of relaxation.

5. Repeat this sequence with the same group, but use only about half the tension.

6. Repeat again with the same muscle group, but allow little movement so that only slight tension can be detected.

For the muscle groups of the lower limbs, trunk, and face it is only necessary to tense the muscles once, very slightly—just enough to recognize the tension. Then let it slide away. Feel the difference. Notice the pleasant warmth of relaxation.

Muscle Groups	**Tension Reducing Exercises**
1. Dominant hand	Lift hand and make a fist; relax.
Other hand	Lift hand and make a fist; relax.
2. Dominant arm	Lift arm at shoulder; relax.
Other arm	Lift arm at shoulder; relax.
3. Shoulders	Shrug shoulders; relax.

Repeat each of the above three times with progressively less tension.

4. Right foot	Bend toes, relax; lift toes, relax.
Left foot	Bend toes, relax; lift toes, relax.
5. Right leg	Start to bend knee (drag heel up slightly); relax.
Left leg	Start to bend knee (drag heel up slightly); relax.
6. Buttocks	Squeeze together; relax.
7. Abdomen	Make abdomen tight and hard; relax.
8. Chest and neck	Squeeze shoulder blades together and slightly arch back, pressing head backward; relax.
9. Breathing	Take a slow deep breath and relax completely as you exhale. Repeat two or three times.
10. Upper face and scalp	Raise eyebrows; relax. Close eyes tightly; relax.

11. Centre face	Scowl and wrinkle nose; relax. Widen cheeks and brows; relax.
12. Lower face	Purse lips; relax. Smile; relax. Drop jaw; relax.
13. Breathing	Take a slow deep breath and relax completely as you exhale. Repeat two or three times.

One can also try certain yogic *asanas* such as meditation or *dhyana* for better effect.

Technique for Progressive Relaxation of the Whole Body

1. Tense all the muscles together and hold for five seconds.

2. Feel the tension, notice it carefully, then release. Let all the tension slide away.

3. Notice any remaining tension. Release it.

4. Take a deep breath. Say "relax" softly to yourself as you breathe out slowly.

5. Remain totally relaxed.

6. Repeat breathing in and out slowly, saying "relax," staying perfectly relaxed.

7. Do this three times.

8. The exercise has ended — enjoy the relaxation.

For people with very painful joints, the technique may not be the best exercise for relaxation. If it causes any pain, the pain may distract from the relaxation. If this is the case for you, try the following techniques.

Four Basic Elements

A Quiet Environment: *Turn off* not only iternal stimuli but also distractions.

An Object to Dwell Upon or a Mental device: For example repeating a word or sound like the word *one,* gazing at a symbol like a flower, or concentrating on a feeling, such as peace.

A Passive Attitude: This is the most essential factor. It is an emptying of all thoughts and distractions from your mind. Thoughts, imagery, and feeling may drift into awareness—don't concentrate on them, but allow them to pass on.

A Comfortable Position: You should be comfortable enough to remain in the same position for 20 minutes.

Technique for Eliciting the Relaxation Response

1. Sit quietly in a comfortable position.

2. Close your eyes.

3. Deeply relax all your muscles, beginning at your feet and progressing up to your face. Keep them relaxed.

4. Breathe in through your nose. Become aware of your breathing. As you breathe out through your mouth, say the word *one* silently to yourself. Try to empty all thoughts from your mind, concentrate on *one*.

5. Continue for 10 to 20 minutes—you may open your eyes to check the time, but do not use an alarm. When you finish, sit quietly for several minutes, at first with your eyes closed. Do not stand up for a few minutes.

6. Do not worry about whether you are successful in achieving a deep level of relaxation. Maintain a passive attitude and permit relaxation to occur at its own pace. When distracting thoughts occur, try to ignore them by not dwelling upon them, and return to repeating *one*.

7. Practice once or twice daily, but ideally not within two hours after any meal, since digestive processes seem to interfere with elicitation of relaxation responses.

You may have noticed that this exercise is very much like meditation. In fact, meditation has provided the principles of the relaxation response. There is no need to spend a lot of money to learn to meditate. You now know all the steps.

Self-Massage

Self-massage is also a relaxation technique which helps manage arthritis. It has many benefits, such as release of tension, preparation of the body for exercise by relaxing muscles and joints and increase in blood circulation throughout the body. Self-massaging also provides comforting heat and warmth to an affected joint.The techniques and procedures of self-massaging are simple. One can do them without any equipment at home, at place of work or even while waiting for the bus. Massage with baby oil can help your hands move smoothly over the skin, but oil is not at all necessary. It can be done without even removing your clothes.

The techniques of self-massage include:

1. Kneading, as if you were preparing dough to bake in the oven;

2. Deep pressure in firm circular motions; and

3. Firm pressure with fingertips pressing deeply into the muscles. You can combine these techniques to gain the desired relaxation in your joints.

Now, all you need to do is explore and experiment to find the area of tension and the proper technique for release and relaxation. Try self-massage on your neck, back, shoulders, legs, feet and fingers.

These and other varieties of relaxation (such as hypnosis, self-hypnosis, biofeedback, and autogenic training) are not scientifically proven treatments for arthritis, and we make no special claims for them. Many individuals in our classes report substantial benefit from these practices, however, and we feel that they have merit for some if used as an adjunct to and not a substitute for a sound basic programme.

A Word of Caution: Various relaxation techniques are often sold in expensive packages as a cure-all for almost everything. Such expensive courses are not necessary. If you want to take a relaxation course, check the following points to avoid unnecessary expense and disappointment.

1. Is the course offered by a reputable institution?

2. Is the cost reasonable?

3. Are any claims or promises made for a cure? If so, look elsewhere.

Hugs and Kisses

Feeling loved and needed by others is important to all of us. Even though the capabilities of people with arthritis may be reduced, family members and friends must not dwell on their deficiencies but should stress their remaining capabilities and encourage them to use them. At such times extra affection, caring, and touching can be supportive and reassuring.

Sexual relationships can be maintained even though one partner has a physical discomfort. Physicians and therapists have suggestions for many people whose diseases temporarily interfere with happy relationships. For example, some people benefit by trying different positions for sexual intercourse that avoid placing weight or stress on uncomfortable joints. Some find that having sexual intercourse early in the morning or during the day is better than in the evening when they are fatigued. Sometimes a warm bath or shower before intercourse relaxes sore joints and muscles and makes the participant more receptive to arousal and response.

Techniques that make sexual relationships more enjoyable for non-arthritis sufferers work for individuals with arthritis, too. For example, gentle caresses, back rubs, and overall body massage may enrich a sexual experience. Also, carefully placed pillows and a comfortable bed that is large enough to permit a variety of positions may be helpful.

If you have questions about your sexual activity, discuss them with your physician or physical therapist. They are accustomed to talking about this subject and will reassure you that your concerns are shared by many others who have found good solutions to some of the same questions.

Maintaining an intimate, caring relationship can provide a source of strength and reassurance.

9

Women, Children and Arthritis

If you are female, you are more likely to have arthritis than if you are male. Scientists can't explain why this happens, but they do know that, of the 31 million adults and children in the United States who have some form of arthritis, more than 20 million are women. About 250,000 children have juvenile rheumatoid arthritis, and of those, more girls than boys are affected.

Women and Arthritis

Some women develop arthritis in their early 20's or at a younger age. Rheumatoid arthirits is the most serious type; if left untreated, it can lead to permanent joint deformities, disability, and damage to the body's vital organs.

In many cases of rheumatoid arthritis, symptoms decrease during pregnancy but sometimes flare up again after delivery. The manifestations of systemic lupus erythematosus (SLE) may become worse during pregnancy. Researchers suspect that natural hormonal changes in the female body play a role but that hormones are not the entire answer. Researchers are working on this puzzle and hope to have more answers as knowledge about arthritis increases. Meanwhile, many health care professionals are exploring the unique effects of arthritis on women. Study projects focus on emotional and physical manifestations of the disease, pain and depression, developing positive mental attitudes, coping and change, mothering, dependency, and physical appearance.

The US Arthritis Foundation advises all women to be aware of the warning signs of arthritis and to seek early diagnosis and prompt, proper treatment. The warning signs are:

1. Persistent pain and stiffness on arising
2. Pain or swelling in one or more joints
3. Tingling sensation in fingertips, hands or feet
4. Unexplained weight loss, fever, anaemia, or fatigue

Having any one or more of these signs does not necessarily mean that you have arthritis, but if you do, you should have a check-up and obtain a diagnosis.

You *CAN* Remain Active: If you do have arthritis, you can preserve your active lifestyle with individualized treatment including medication, special exercises, rest, self-help aids for daily activities and possibly surgery. You can learn to live with the illness and continue to lead a normal life with minimal discomfort by following several guidelines:

1. Follow your doctor's advice. Take medications as prescribed. Do the exercises recommended and take rest periods.

2. Don't rely on self-medication, fad diets, or quack remedies.

3. Avoid being overweight. Eat properly. Avoid being overtired.

4. Don't be rigid in your standards at home. If you have to stop a household chore before completion because you are tired, rest and come back to it later.

5. Talk frankly with your family about your disease and the limitations it places on you.

6. Encourage participation in household chores by other family members so that you can rest when necessary.

7. Don't encourage family members to pamper you just because you have arthritis.

8. Seek out special exercise groups for women with arthritis. Learn as much as you can about your disease by keeping up with new developments through literature and other media.

The Arthritic Child: Special Role of Parents

If you are the parent of an arthritic child, you and the child's physician must become partners in providing care for the child. Your role will include providing the emotional support, the chronically ill child needs, as well as helping the child follow the physician's programme of medication, rest and exercise. Children with arthritis need encouragement to grow and develop emotionally and socially as well as physically.

Understanding Juvenile Rheumatoid Arthritis

The most common form of arthritis in children is juvenile rheumatoid arthritis. Many children with the disease have remissions and recurrences. Some children experience little or no permanent damage as they grow. Yet in some cases there are serious complications in the form of eye disease and even blindness. Early and proper diagnosis is essential to prevent complications.

Juvenile rheumatoid arthritis may begin with a high fever, rash, and a *sick-all-over* feeling. It can affect the heart, liver, and spleen and chiefly affects joints in the fingers, ankles, knees, elbows, hips, and feet, causing inflammation, pain and some degree of immobility.

Juvenile rheumatoid arthritis is sometimes called a *hidden handicap*. A child may show few outward signs of disease because the damage and pain are inside the body. In some cases, however, the damage interferes with normal growth. A child may be small for her or his age, have a receding lower jaw, walk with a stiff gait, or have some joint deformity in the wrists and fingers.

Treatment: Each case of juvenile rheumatoid arthritis is unique and what the doctor recommends for each child depends on the severity and pattern of the disease, the age of the girl or boy, and what joints and other parts of the body are affected.

Treatment may require a long time and may include medication, frequent eye examinations, heat treatments, rest and special exercises, splints to be worn at certain times, and possibly surgery. A variety of antiinflammatory drugs is used. Aspirin is the most frequently prescribed medication for juvenile rheumatoid arthritis because it reduces inflammation in the joints and relieves pain. To get the best results from aspirin, some children with arthritis must regularly take large doses, even after pain and inflammation have subsided. Youngsters vary in their tolerance for aspirin, and parents should be sure that they are administering aspirin to their children only as prescribed and under the guidance of their physician.

In some cases the youngster with arthritis may be advised to go to a hospital for special tests. Otherwise, most children with arthritis are kept at home with their families, go to school and participate in social activities as much as possible.

Physicians say the outlook for those with rheumatoid arthritis that begins in childhood is often better than for those who get the disease as adults.

Exercise and Physical Therapy: If your child has rheumatoid arthritis, your child's physician and physical therapist have probably instructed you about exercising the child's joints to keep them mobile, improve their functioning, and prevent or minimize disabilities. Usually such exercises are done at home in the mornings and evenings.

Your child may have to get up a little earlier than others to allow time to loosen up before school. Often the most severe discomfort is in the early morning, and the duration of the stiffness is an indication of the severity of the disease. It may last longer on some days than on others. Starting the day with a warm bath is effective for many children.

Taking Medication in School: If your child takes medication for arthritis, even aspiritn, his or her teacher should be advised. Schools vary in their procedures. Some prefer that medications, be kept by teachers or the school nurse. You may want to ask the teacher to cooperate so that the child does not have to make several trips a day to a special office at medication time. Also subtle supervision by the teacher during the course of the day may be necessary so that the child does not intentionally *forget* to take medication in an effort to appear just like the other children.

Being One of the Kids: At times your child may wear a plastic or metal splint on an arm, wrist, or hand to rest inflamed joints and keep them in the proper position to prevent or correct deformities. If this is necessary, you may want to explain the function of these splints to the teacher so that correct information can be given to the other children and to remove the mysterious air from your child's appearance.

Activity is one of the best medicines for a child with arthritis because it makes the child feel like other children. Moreover, exercise helps reduce joint stiffness. However, the arthritic child should be encouraged not to overexert during strenuous activities that may cause more inflammation. Although a child can go to school during a flare-up of the arthritis, some limitations should be placed on physical activities in the classroom and playground at those times.

Making Each Day Easier: Children with arthritis may benefit from suggestions for coping with everyday situations. For example, they may sometimes have difficulty in carrying schoolbooks and lunch trays, turning door handles, flushing toilets, turning on water faucets, writing fast enough to complete tests during the allotted time, opening lockers, writing on blackboards or raising a hand to ask a question. Many of the self-help aids available for adults can be adapted for use by youngsters. For details see Chapter 12.

Young people with arthritis find a variety of ways to overcome difficulties. For example, some students keep one set of books at home and another at school so that books do not have to be carried each day. Some use a shoulder bag or backpack to avoid putting stress on hands and wrists. Others enlist a group of buddies to assist routinely with specific difficult tasks. When children understand each other's limitations they are generally eager and willing to help without making the afflicted child feel different and uncomfortable.

You can help by advising your child's teacher that long periods of sitting can make the pain and stiffness of arthritis worse. The teacher might help by occasionally asking the child to perform some chore involing movement, such as collecting papers from the class. If there is difficulty in walking fast enough from one room to another, the child might be excused a few minutes earlier than the other children. In a multistorey school building, the child might be permitted to use an elevator to prevent undue stress on leg joints while climbing stairs.

Your Child's Future

Although current treatments are effective for many children, much remains to be learned about juvenile rheumatiod arthritis. As more is learned about possible causes, better treatments can be initiated earlier. Your physician keeps up to date on developments as they occur and will advise you when better medications are available or when changes in your child's treatment plan are necessary.

To serve the special needs of young arthritis patients and their families, the US Arthritis Foundation has established a membership section called the American Juvenile Arthritis Organization. Parents, patients, relatives, friends, teachers, and health professionals are invited to join. Through this organization you can learn about additional association that provide information, assurance, and assistance. For details see Chapter 12.

10

The Cost of Arthritis

Arthritis hurts. It is also expensive. In financial terms the overall costs to the world economy run into hundreds of billions of dollars. In human terms—pain, suffering, and disability—the costs cannot be measured.

Arthritis takes its toll in reduced quality of life for many families and for many individuals. For business and industry it is a costly factor due to absenteeism, loss of productivity, and disability payments. It is the leading cause of industrial absenteeism and is second only to heart disease as a reason for disability payments. It is the nation's number one crippling disease.

For many individuals delays in receiving professional care mean additional personal and societal costs. Early diagnosis and prompt, appropriate treatment can cut costs. To business, successful treatment of arthritis can mean a reduction of both human suffering and economic loss. Only as more people become knowledgeable about the warning signs of arthritis and the importance of professional treatment at an early stage of the disease can the upward spiralling of arthritis-related costs be reduced.

An Expensive Disease

If you have arthritis, you have felt the costs. Other taxpayers, employers, insurance companies, government, and health-related associations also have felt the costs. More than 31 million Americans have one of the 100 or more different forms of arthritis requiring medical care, and more than 1 million new victims join the ranks each year. Acording to the US Arthritis Foundation, the direct and indirect annual costs to the national economy due to arthritis, run to billions of dollars in the US alone, including lost wages and medical bills.

Estimates indicate that one in seven people, or one in every three families, has arthritis. Osteoarthritis has claimed about 16 million, and more than 250,000 children have one of several forms of arthritis. Of those the National Centre for Health Statistics of the US says that more than 7.3 million people are disabled as a result of arthritis and contribute to the total of 525 million days of restricted activity each year in that country. Arthritis accounts for more than $1 billion in annual disability payments, or about 15 percent of all Social Security disability insurance payments in the United States. Of the $5 billion spent annually on medical care, nearly $1 billion is spent on quack remedies and unproven drugs and devices.

The Costs of Quackery

Because there is still no cure for arthritis, many sufferers fall prey to fast talkers promoting quack remedies. According to the US Arthritis Foundation, arthritis victims spend about $ 1 billion a year on remedies and devices that do no good and in some cases do considerable harm. Buying and using quack remedies is merely a waste of money for some. For others there are more serious consequences. Persons using unproven remedies delay or reject medically prescribed therapy. The US Arthritis Foundation says that the average arthritis patient waits more than four years after noticing symptoms to seek appropriate medical care. Some people wait even longer because they try remedies for self-treatment. Some self-treatment remedies may be harmful because the indivdual's overall health condition, allergies, and other medications are not taken into consideration. There may be side-effects of the so-called quick cures. In more recent years quack remedies have ranged from copper bracelets to soaking up radiation from uranium in abandoned mines. Many food fads and exotic drugs have been touted. Food fads have included cod liver oil, sea water, extracts from shellfish, and many others. The US Arthritis Foundation says that no food or vitamin has been shown to affect arthritis, either as a cause or as a cure (with exceptions, in some cases, for gouty arthritis).

Quackery continues to flourish despite efforts of the US Arthritis Foundation and major medical centres, which warn against unproven remedies. Because arthritis is a disease that tends to come and go in many individuals, some think they are being cured when their disease goes into remission in its natural course. Some think they feel better just because they are taking something new. This is a placebo effect. While there is no real change in the condition, the person may feel better temporarily simply because he or she wants to.

Recognizing Quack Remedies, Devices and Clinics

How can you tell if a remedy is appropriate for your arthritis? Can you determine whether a clinic is reputable? Be wary of any claims of cures. As of now there is no cure for arthritis. When there is one, your doctor will know about it. Be wary of claims that one miracle drug, device, or treatment will cure all forms of arthritis or other pain. Arthritis takes many forms and requires individualized treatment.

Start with your family doctor, who knows you and your health history. Your own physician will prescribe a treatment plan that will include proven therapies, such as medication, rest, exercise, perhaps losing weight, a nutritious diet, and a healthy lifestyle. In some cases physicians refer arthritis patients to arthritis specialists called *rheumatologists* for treatment. Rheumatologists do not advertise and receive most of their patients on a referral basis from reputable physicians. If your physician advises you to go to a rheumatologist, you can be sure that you will receive appropriate treatment for your disease.

If your have any doubt about a course of treatment prescribed for you, consult another doctor. No reputable physician will mind having a consultation by another specialist who will give a second opinion.

Education Will Dispel Myths and Save Money

Many people mistakenly think they can treat arthritis effectively themselves by using advertised remedies or devices. Public education about arthritis may help offset the thriving quackery business and prevent needless waste of money. As more people learn more about arthritis fewer will be vulnerable to unproven remedies.

According to the US Arthritis Foundation, Americans have five major misconceptions about arthritis. They say that people generally have more misinformation about arthritis than any other common disease. Because wrong information can be harmful and costly, it is important to understand the facts.

Arthritis is not a Serious Disease: While it is true that many people have minor aches and pains that they think are symptoms of rheumatism or arthritis, arthritis can also be serious and crippling or life-threatening. In some cases, arthritis patients are seriously ill. Some have deformed hands, wrists, knees, feet, and hips. Others may suffer damage to vital organs such as the kidneys, heart, and brain. With proper treatment, however, these effects can be prevented or offset. It is wrong to believe that arthritis is not a serious disease.

Self-diagnosis and Self-treatment Work for Arthritis: You can't determine what kind of arthritis you have. Different kinds require different treatment. While you experiment wth unproven remedies, you can dangerously damage your joints. Medicines you might take without medical supervision can also have serious side effects. It is dangerous to believe that self-diagnosis and self-treatment work for arthritis.

Doctors can't do Much for Arthritis: Much can be done to prevent the crippling effects of arthritis. Damage to joints can be reduced or corrected in many cases. Damage to vital organs can be arrested or reversed. Medications are available for the control of pain. Combinations of medications, rest and exercise work for many people. Getting an early diagnosis and proper medical care before joints are irreversibly damaged can prevent the serious effects of arthritis.

Arthritis is Mostly an Old People's Disease: Many people have had arthritis since they were relatively young. Some forms of arthritis can start in infancy. Most, however, begin during adulthood. It is not true that arthritis is an old people's disease.

Diet is Important in Arthritis: Physicians once cautioned people with gouty arthritis about certain foods, but today appropriate medications have given even gouty arthritis sufferers more freedom of choice concerning foods. For details see Chapter 7. Special diets and fad foods do not relieve arthritis. The US Arthritis Foundation advises that nothing you eat will cause or aggravate arthritis. However, malnutrition or excess weight *can* worsen the course of the disease.

Saving Money and Days

To the individual, improved understanding about the nature of arthritis and effective treatment for the disease can save money and result in a better quality of life. To employers, better knowledge of the possibilities of controlling arthritis can mean keeping people on the payroll and off the compensation rolls. For family life, better understanding and therapies can mean continuing happy, normal relationships. Financial and emotional savings can be realized from many directions.

If you or someone you care about has arthritis, you can save money and work toward continuing productivity by learning more about the nature of the disease. You can keep up with developments as they occur in research. You can obtain information to help make life easier. Many organizations, nationally and locally, make available services and products that can help you reduce the costs of arthritis by enabling you to continue your lifestyle in as normal and productive a way as possible. Some of these resources are utlined in Chapter 12.

11

What's the Future for You?

If you have received treatment for your arthritis, you may already have benefited from advances made within the past few years. While no cure has been discovered for most forms of arthritis, many recent improvements in treatment may relieve pain, prevent deformity, and make it possible for you and many others to lead more normal lives.

Increased public awareness of arthritis has helped focus attention on the need for research and the many advantages of improving therapy. Each year scientists uncover more missing pieces to the arthritis puzzle. Hundreds of drugs as well as other treatments now are in experimental stages that might soon do even more to help ease the pain and disability associated with arthritis. Researchers are excited about many future possibilities because of scientific projects currently under way.

Learning More about Causes

In efforts to find better treatments, scientists are seeking a better understanding of the complex set of diseases known as arthritis. To do that, many researchers are studying functions of the basic cells and processes that keep the human body in good working order.

As briefly mentioned in Chapter 2, some forms of arthritis

are believed to be caused by a defect in the body's immune system. When the immune system works correctly, the body is able to recognize antigens as foreign invaders (such as viruses and bacteria) and fight them off with inflammation. When the system is defective, in addition to recognizing and fighting off the antigens, the body's defender cells may also attack normal body tissues, causing damage and pain. This knowledge has led researchers to one possible course of action. Understanding how the immune mechanism works will help you understand what they are trying to do.

Soon after an antigen enters the body it meets the recognition cells of the immune system. The monocyte is a cell that transforms the antigen so that it can be identified by the lymphocyte. Lymphocytes distinguish between normal substances in the body and those that are foreign. There are two types of lymphocytes: T-lymphocytes and B-lymphocytes. When they work properly, B-lymphocytes change into larger cells known as *plasma cells,* which manufacture antibodies that attach themselves to the antigen and form a *complex. Complement,* a series of blood proteins, is activated by this complex. To finish the job of killing off the antigen the activated complement attracts cells called *phagocytes*. Phagocytes engulf the complex, and their enzymes work to "digest" and destroy the complex. T-lymphocytes may directly attack and destroy and antigen and also produce substances that stimulate or suppress other lymphocytes.

Researchers know that the lymphocytes in individuals with rheumatoid arthritis behave differently from normal lymphocytes. Research efforts have demonstrated that some patients with rheumatoid arthritis improve temporarily when large numbers of these lymphocytes are removed from their blood. Because of this knowledge, researchers hope to develop a more direct treatment against the defective lymphocytes.

Genetics

Recent evidence indicates that abnormalities of the immune system may be inherited or are genetic in nature. The discovery of human leukocyte antigens (HLA) could provide an important breakthrough, not only for arthritis sufferers but also for victims of other diseases, such as multiple sclerosis, some types of diabetes, and some types of leukemia. HLAs are a series of proteins on the surface of body cells that are determined by inheritance; the proteins on a person's cells are inherited from his or her parents. Certain HLA proteins are present more frequently in individuals with certain forms of arthritis, suggesting that the tendency to develop some forms of arthritis may be inherited.

Some dramatic evidence that heredity plays a vital role in the development of many types of arthritis came during 1990 from the University of Texas Southwestern Medical Center and The Howard Hughes Medical Institute in Dallas, Texas. Researchers inserted two human genes into fertilized rat eggs, where the genes became part of the animals' own genetic code. The two genes, which have been linked to a group of arthritic diseases (ankylosing spondylitis, inflammatory arthritis, and arthritis associated with psoriasis and certain conditions associated with inflammation of the bowel), are identified as HLA-B27 and human beta-2 microglobulin. Together they produce a protein produce called B27. However, it remains to be determined exactly how the protein causes arthritic disorders.

The B27 is one of a number of molecules referred to as human lymphocyte antigens, which help regulate the white blood cells of the body's immune defence system.

Researchers believed that these genes have long been the markers for some arthritis diseases, but were suprised to see the animals with the transplanted genes develop significant symptoms. However, mice transplanted with the human genes did not develop arthritic diseases. Estimates are that 7 to 8 percent of people worldwide carry the two genes and that their risk of developing an arthritic disease is one to 20 percent.

Additionally, a gene has been found in certain families that leads to increased risk of osteoarthritis because it causes a defect in the cartilage. Researchers hope that in the future, this gene

145

can be modified and the defect corrected, thereby decreasing the risk of osteoarthritis in these people.

Better treatments for arthritis will become available as researchers develop more links between arthiritis and genetics.

Thus the immune system with a genetic (inherited) tendency seems to be at work in some forms of arthritis. However, there still must be an unspecified trigger that sparks the chain reaction of self-detructive immune reactions leading to arthritis. Many researchers are trying to discover the identity of the antigens that trigger the immune system.

Viruses

Recent research has indicated that viruses may be the trigger for some types of arthritis. Certain viruses can lie dormant in the body for long periods. The suspected arthritis virus may be dormant and then become active and activate the body's immune system. Somehow the virus tricks the lymphocytes, and, in addition to attacking the virus, the immune system attacks the body tissue itself. This starts a destructive chain reaction, and the virus slips away, undetected, possibly settling in another part of the body to do more damage.

One virus that may be involved in the arthritis process has been identified as the Epstein Barr virus (EBV). This is the same virus responsible for infectious mononucleosis. By the time most people are 30 years old they have the EBV antibodies (elements the body has produced to fight off the EBV) in their blood. This means that the EBV at one time infected them but their systems effectively fought it off without any symptoms of diseases appearing. While not proven, some scientists suspect that the presence of the EBV, perhaps combined with an inherited suceptibility, may lead to rheumatoid arthritis.

Bacteria

Bacteria are more complex organisms than viruses. Some forms or arthritis, called *infectious arthritis,* are caused by direct bacterial infection of the joint. Early diagnosis of a bacterial joint infection is critical since infectious arthritis can be cured by the administration of antibiotics that kill the bacteria before the joint is damaged permanently.

Researchers have evidence that bacteria can also indirectly trigger arthritic disease. One example is the arthritis developing in some patients after intestinal bypass operations. This form of arthritis appears to be caused by bacteria that would normally be expelled from the body through the bowel, now escaping from the shortened intestine and slipping into the bloodstream. The bacteria trigger the immune system and trick it into attacking body tissue. One form of *bypass arthritis* closely resembles rhumatoid arthritis.

Bacteria may also indirectly trigger another form of arthritis known as *Reiter's syndrome*. In 1962 an epidemic of bacterial dysentery occurred among the crew members of the U.S. Navy cruiser Little Rock. Out of the hundreds of sailors affected by diarrhea, 10 subsequently developed Reiter's syndrome. The solution to this puzzle was found 15 years later when it was discovered that some of the men who developed Reiter's syndrome carried the genetic marker known as HLA B27 on their cells. Therefore, it appears that the bacteria was the trigger for Reiter's syndrome only in those men who were genetically predisposed.

New Treatments for Arthritis

While research has made great strides in furthering our understanding of arthritis, there still is no cure for most forms of arthritis. Therefore, the best treatment programme for arthritis must make use of all available therapies – rest and exercise, physical therapy, proper nutrition, medication, and surgery when indicated. Thus while medications are a basic part of arthritis therapy, they should never be used as the sole treatment.

Nonsteroidal Antiinflammatory Drugs (NSAIDs)

Aspirin is still the most commonly utilized NSAID. It is the least expensive, most readily obtained, and most effective therapy for many forms of arthritis. Aspirin should always be taken with meals or a snack to minimize side effects on the stomach.

However, many patients still cannot tolerate aspirin in doses high enough to treat arthritis. In this situation the other NSAIDs have been very useful. NSAIDs such as naproxen, tolemetin sodium, indomethacin, ibuprofen, sulindac, and others are as effective as aspirin but have fewer side effects. In addition the newer longer acting NSAIDs need only be taken once or twice daily for maximum effectiveness.

Immunosuppressants

An Important group of drugs known as *immunosuppressants* is expected to play a bigger role in arthritis therapy if the associated side effects can be controlled. Immunosuppressant drugs can help check the activity of the immune system. These drugs are both strong and dangerous, and researchers are constantly striving to develop immunosuppressants with fewer serious side effects. Immunosuppressants such as azathioprine, cyclophosphamide, chlorambucil, and methotrexate are commonly used to modify the chain of events that leads to inflammation of joints.

Immunostimulants

Another experimental drug is an immunostimulant known as *levamisole*. This drug has the reverse action of the immunosuppressants and it is unclear why and how it works. Although it opens the possibility of a new approach to arthritis treatment, researchers emphasize that it is still in highly experimental stages.

Surgical Treatment

Recent advances in surgical treatment for arthritis are outlined in Chapter 5. For more than 30 years, doctors have been performing an operation called *synovectomy* to remove inflamed tissue from joints of rheumatoid arthritis patients. Drawbacks of the procedure were that diseased tissues could be left behind and the tissue frequently grew back after the operation. Also, the period of recovery was long and involved a lengthy period of physical therapy.

Now, with the aid of a recently developed device called an *arthroscope*, the performance of synovectomy is easier and more effective. The arthroscope is an optical instrument about the size of a pencil. The arthroscopist looks into a joint through the device, locates diseased tissues, assesses damage, and inserts another instrument through the tube to extract the diseased tissue and eroded cartilage. With this device, arthroscopists can remove synovial membranes from areas behind the knee that are usually inaccessible during routine arthrotomies. Arthroscopy is a shorter procedure with less bleeding than arthrotomy. Each incision is closed with just one stitch, and there is less potential for complications. It appears that many arthritis sufferers in the future may benefit from this new technique.

Radiation Therapy

Radiation therapy has worked for a very few patients in experimental situations. Researchers theorize that radiation kills some blood cells and thus reduces the lymphocyte activity that leads to inflammation. In a recent study at Stanford University, of 11 persons with rheumatoid arthritis in whom conventional treatments did not produce relief, nine experienced *significant response* to radiation therapy.

Treatment by Blood Filtration

Major research efforts are directed toward looking at factors in the blood that are believed to be involved in the development of arthritis and specifically in the development of rheumatoid arthritis and systemic lupus erythematosus (SLE).

A recent approach to treating arthritis in some research centres has involved replacing certain components of the blood. Immune factors battling body tissue cause debris that builds up in the blood and leads to inflammtion associated with arthritis. For several years researchers have experimented with a process called *plasmapheresis*. In this process some of the patients's plasma is removed and replaced with fresh donor plasma. Plasmapherisis has produced varying results in patients. However, the limited supply of donor plasma, along with the high cost of replacing the blood supply several times a week over a period of weeks, made plasmapheresis impractical for a disease as widespread as arthritis.

Randall S. Krakauer, MD, head of an arthritis research team at the Cleveland Clinic Foundation, Cleveland, Ohio, summed up some of the problems involved with plasmapheresis: "Our best information is that it is effective in the treatment of rheumatoid arthritis and it is incredibly expensive. Most of the cost is in blood donor proteins. We generate 4 million units of donor blood in the United States each year. There are 7 million people with rheumatoid arthritis. It's just not possible to do plasmapheresis on very many."

Now a newer process, based on plasmapheresis, may hold more promise. Called *selective apheresis,* the process removes the blood and, instead of replacing it with new blood, filters it through an elaborate machine somewhat similar to a kidney dialysis machine. The blood is cleaned of possibly detrimental substances and then returned to the patient. While the proces is costly, it prevents the additional expense of scarce donor blood.

According to Dr. Krakauer, after a series of selective apheresis treatments termed *cryofiltration,* the majority of patients tested experienced remissions or marked improvement in their conditions. Some remissions lasted up to several months. Because results with apheresis have been so encouraging, researchers believe the process will soon move out of the experiemental stage into approved usage. The clinical trials of the technique were directed by the Cleveland Clinic's team at several major health centres in the United States and Canada. Data from Tokyo and Munich have been consistent with data obtained by the Cleveland Clinic researchers and their affiliates.

Dr. Krakauer speculates that adaptations of the apheresis technique may apply to other diseases. "We call it extra-corporeal therapy," he says. "We hope to develop an immunochemical sorbent to remove from the body what we perceive as abnormal. This is theoretically possible, perhaps in a number of years."

The Need for Continued Research

Eventual control of arthritis must come through better understanding of its causes. In the United States, major research efforts are channelled through the US Arthritis Foundation, which provides grants to selected centres of patient care, research, and training. More than one-third of the total income of the national office is directed toward research. Recipients of the research awards work in more than 50 institutions throughout the United States. The US Arthritis Foundation is the only national voluntary health association devoted exclusively to finding the causes of and cures for all the various form of arthritis.

Researchers know that major efforts are necessary to continue arthritis research. William J. Arnold, MD, Director of Rheumatology at Lutheran General Hospital, Park Ridge, Illinois, summed up the viewpoint of many at a recent meeting of the Illinois chapter of the US Arthritis Foundation: "Federal funding to deal with categorical disease problems should be at a level commensurate with their toll in human terms, coupled with their impact on the national economy. Arthritis currently affects more than 31 million Americans and annually costs the nation $14.5 billion. We have first-rate basic science research going on. There's no other way to get answers. We cannot limit our focus. We are too close to important discoveries."

Public Education: Key to Future Health

In the future, popular attitudes toward health will play a part in relief from the sometimes crippling effects of arthritis. As more people recognize that their lifestyle affects their health, more will recognize that they are to a great extent responsible for the state of their own health. What they eat and drink, whether they smoke, and how they exercise, rest and relax is largely their own decision. People are taking an active role in promoting their own good health through lifestyle changes.

When a disease such as arthritis strikes, many people will make use of the educational and informational services of organizations such as the US Arthritis Foundation. Information is available to help them locate appropriate medical assistance and to cope with the practicalities of everyday life in a more constructive, optimistic manner.

More people are realizing that they need not wait for a miracle cure for relief but can actively pursue better health in many ways. In addition to following the advice of their physician and health care team, they can win the battle with their disease through appropriate rest and exercise, a good, well-balanced diet and overall better physical condition. Techniques for rehabilitation therapy are expanding every day. The interdisciplinary activities of physical therapy, occupational therapy, psychology and psychiatry, together with medicine and surgery, continue to provide help and hope for more people with arthritis each year.

Fewer people now believe in myths and magic relating to arthritis, and more are seeking legitimate treatment and professional care at earlier stages, when treatment may prevent more extensive and possibly permanent joint damage.

Public education programmes are being carried out and more people are benefiting from the latest knowledge about arthritis. Self-help groups, organized by many hospitals and medical centres treating arthritic patients, provide the group support and interchange of information that helps many people with arthritis, face each day. Psychologists say these groups are important to arthritis sufferers because they reinforce physicians' instructions, help to free participants from fear and give each individual the emotional support needed to cope with the disease.

There are many reasons to anticipate better ways of dealing with the problems of arthritis in the future. The keys to developments in arthritis care will come through a combination of improved drugs and increased attention to the interaction between medication and the patient's lifestyle. The future will have much to offer arthritis patients.

12

Resources

Your physician, particularly the rheumatologist, will be your primary source of information about arthritis. Your local hospital or community health centres and the US Arthritis Foundation are other major sources of health education, information on patient groups, self-help aids and equipment.

The US Arthritis Foundation

The US Arthritis Foundation was formed about 40 years ago and is a voluntarily supported organization woking to solve the serious problems associated with all forms of arthritis. Within the Arthritis Foundation are two professional associations : the American Rheumatism Association Section, the world's largest professional society of rheumatologists; and the Arthritis Health Professional Section, whose members are physical and occupational therapists, medical personnel and social workers, and others concerned with arthritis patient care.

The Foundation's major purposes are to support research to prevent and cure all forms of arthritis and to provide professional and public education. Through grants, the Foundation enables many health professionals to work in leading research institutions. With the help of more than 70 chapters throughout the United States the Arthritis Foundation supports community health services for arthritis sufferers.

You can get more information about the Arthritis Foundation by writing to :

Arthritis Foundation

1314 Spring St., NW Atlanta, GA 30309, U.S.A.

Additionally, the American Juvenile Arthritis Organization is for people interested in childhood arthritis.

Indian Rheumatism Association (IRA)

The Indian Rheumatism Association has been quite active ever since 1990 when it was founded. The arthritis health professionals and rheumatologists such as Dr. P.D. Gulati, Prof. (Mrs.) S. Sachdev and Prof. G.G. Mansharamani are of great help to those who need professional guidance.

IRA H.Q.
PD Hinduja Hospital
Medical Research Centre, Bombay

IRA Hyderabad Branch
Nizam Institute of Medical Sciences, Hyderabad

IRA Delhi Branch
213, Rouse Avenue, N. Delhi-110002

IRA Madras Branch
Madras Medical College, Madras

IRA Calcutta Branch
Calcutta Medical College, Calcutta

Other Self-Help Groups

Many groups, organizations, and telephone networks have developed in many countries because persons with similar afflictions or concerns joined together to provide mutual assistance. Individuals with diseases such as arthritis have found that they can not always depend on personal resources alone but can remain independent and enjoy a sense of well-being when their resources are supplemented with the help of others. In these groups a professional may be paid from time to time to give a lecture or an informal presentation. There may be minimal costs for participation.

To learn if there are any self-help groups of interest to you locally, ask your physician, contact your local arthritis clinics or hospital.

These agencies would willingly provide free referral services for individuals seeking self-help groups addressing their concerns or requesting information on the development of new groups. You may be interested in groups relating to issues in addition to arthritis. For example, if you are concerned about losing weight, quitting smoking, overcoming depressive illness, or learning more about the psychological aspects of coping with chronic pain, these self-help referral centres can direct you.

Home Care

Your physician or the local arthritis clinic can assist you in obtaining information on receiving care at home. Your doctor may want a physical therapist to show you and your family how to do exercises at home or may want visiting nurses to provide professional nursing care if you are homebound. He can also advise you about where to purchase orthopaedic equipment and self-help devices for use at home.

Self-Help Equipment

Self-help devices can be purchased, made at home, or adapted for many purposes. The U.S. Arthritis Foundation has published *Self-Help Manual for Arthritis Patients,* Which includes items related to bed, toilet, bath and shower, grooming, dressing, housing, furnishing your home, safety, kitchen planning, meal preparation and eating aids, sewing and needlework aids, communication and vocational aids, travel and shopping, recreation and leisure time, sources for equipment, helpful agencies and organizations, and where to obtain informational literature.

Getting Older

In many communities special services are available for persons who need assistance of various types. Many centres and clubs offer such organized activities and informal socializing for older persons. You may want to contact your local centre for information on what is currently available in your area. One such centre is :

Age Care India Society
J-122, Saket, New Delhi-110 017.

Hospitals & Medical Colleges

Following is a list of some of the many addresses of hospitals & medical colleges in India that also provide assistance and treatment on a local level for persons with arthritis.

Andhra Pradesh

- KEM Hospital, Secundrabad
- King George Hospital, Vishakhapatnam
- Nizam Institute of Medical Sciences, Hyderabad
- Osmania General Hospital, Hyderabad
- Ramnarain Ruia Hospital, Tirupati

Assam

- Assam Medical College & Hospital, Dibrugarh
- Guwahati Medical College & Hospital, Guwahati

Bihar

- Darbhanga Medical College & Hospital, Laheriasarai
- Patna Medical College & Hospital, Patna
- Prince of Wales Medical College & Hospital, Patna
- Rajendra Medical College & Hospital, Ranchi
- R.J.S. Institute of Orthopaedic Rehabilitation & Research Centre, Ranchi

Chandigarh

- PGIMER, Sector-12, Chandigarh

Delhi

- AIIMS, New Delhi.
- Batra Hospital & Medical Research Centre, New Delhi.
- Guru Tegh Bahadur Hospital, Delhi
- Hindu Rao Hospital, Delhi
- LNJP Hospital, New Delhi.
- Moolchand Kharaiti Ram Hospital, New Delhi
- RML Hospiatl, New Delhi
- Safdarjung Hospital, New Delhi
- Sir Ganga Ram Hospital, New Delhi

Gujrat

- B.J. Medical College & Civil Hospital, Ahmedabad
- Central Institute of Research in Indegenous Systems of Medicine, Jamnagar
- Seth V C General Hospital, Ahmedabad
- Shri Sayajirao General Hospital, Vadodara

Goa

- Goa Medical College, Panaji

Himachal Pradesh

- Indira Gandhi Medical College & Hospital, Shimla

Jammu & Kashmir
- Govt. Medical College & Hospital, Jammu

Kerala
- Medical College & Hospital, Trivandrum

Karnataka
- Victoria Hospital, Bangalore
- St.John's Medical College & Hospital, Bangalore

Madhya Pradesh
- Kamla Raja Hospital, Gwalior
- JA Group of Hospitals, Gwalior
- M.G Memorial Medical College & Hospital, Indore
- Ispat General Hospital, Rourkela
- Govt. Medical College Hospital, Jabalpur

Maharashtra
- KEM Hospital, Bombay
- BYL Nair Hospital, Bombay
- PD Hinduja Hospital, Bombay
- Grant Medical College, Bombay
- AFMC Command Hospital, Pune
- Institute of Rehabilitation, Bombay
- Smt. BCJ General Hospital, Bombay
- Jaslok Hospital, Bombay

Manipur
- Regional Medical College & Hospitals, Imphal

Orissa
- S.C.B Medical College & Hospital, Cuttack

Punjab
- Govt. Medical College & S.G.T.B Hospital, Amritsar
- Rajindra Hospital & Govt. Medical College, Patiala

Rajasthan
- Sawai Man Singh Hospital, Jaipur
- Sir Padampat Maternal & Child Institute, Jaipur
- J.L.N Medical College & Hospital, Ajmer

Tamil Nadu
- Govt. Stainley Hospital, Madras
- Christian Medical College & Hospital, Vellore
- Madras Medical College & Govt. General Hospital, Madras
- Govt. Rajaji Hospital, Madurai

Uttar Pradesh
- K.G Medical College & Hospital, Lucknow
- Sir Sunderlal Hospital, BHU, Varanasi
- S.V.B.P Hospital, Meerut
- Sarojani Naidu College & Hospital, Agra
- J.L.N Medical College & Hospital, A.M.U, Aligarh
- Govt. Medical College & Hospital, Kanpur

West Bengal
- Calcutta Medical College, Calcutta
- Institute of PGMER, Calcutta
- School of Tropical Medicine, Calcutta
- National Medical Institute & Hospital, Calcutta

International Organizations

If you have specific questions relating to your arthritis, many organizations may be able to provide answers. The following are a few sources that may be helpful:

American Occupational Therapy Association
6000 Executive Blvd.
Rockville, MD 20852 USA

Architectural and Transportation Barriers Compliance Board
330 C St., SW
Washington, DC 20201 USA

The Arthritis Society
920 Yonge St.
Ste. 420
Toronto, Ontario M5E 1E6 Canada

Rehabilitation International USA
1123 Broadway
New York, NY 10010 USA

Moss Rehabilitation Hospital
Travel Information Center
12th St. and Tabor Rd.
Philadelphia, PA 19141 USA

National Association of the Physically Handicapped, Inc.
76 Elm St.
London, Ohio 43140 USA

National Information Center for the Handicapped
PO Box 1492
Washington, DC 20013 USA

Information Office
National Institutes of Arthritis, Diabetes, and
Kidney Diseases
Bldg. 31, Rm 9A-04, Bethesda, MD 20205 USA

National Safety Council
Dept. H.P.O., Box 11171
Chicago, IL 60611 USA

Public Affairs Committee, Inc. (pamphlet publishers)
381 Park Avenue South
New York, NY 10016 USA

British Rheumatism & Arthritis Association
6, Grosvenor Square, London SW 1

The Arthritis & Rheumatism Council
Faraday House
8/10 Charing Cross Road,
London WC 2.

Periodicals

Following is a list of periodicals of interest to persons with arthritis.

Accent on Living, PO Box 700, Bloomington, IL 61701. Quarterly.

Arthritic Care Research, Vol. 3, pp. 29-35, 1990; The article 'Dance-based Aerobic Exercise for Rheumatoid Arthritis' by S.G. Perlman, K.J. Connell, A. Clark, MS Robinson, P. Conlon, M. Gecht, P. Caldron and J.M. Sinacore is worth reading.

Closer Look, National Information Center for the Handicapped, PO Box 1492, Washington, DC 20013. Free information on topics of interest to persons with disabilities.

Clearinghouse on the Handicapped, Office of Special Education and Rehabilitative Services, Room 3106, Switzer Bldg., 330 C St. SW, Washington, DC 20202.

COPH Bulletin, National Congress of Organizations of the Physically Handicapped. Apt. 203, 2040 Highland Ave., Birmingham, AL 35205.

Disabled USA, The President's Committee on Employment of the Handicapped, Washington, DC 20210.

Encore, National Library Service for the Blind and Physically Handicapped, Library of Congress, Washington, DC 20540. Bi-monthly recording for Talking Books, readers of selections from publications for the disabled.

Health Action, Vol. 2, 1991, PO Box 2153, 157/6 Staff Road, Gunrock Enclave, Secunderabad.

Mainstream : Magazine of the Able-Disabled. 861 6th Ave. Ste. 610, San Diego, CA 92101.

National Rehabilitation Information Center, 4407 Eighth St. NW, Catholic University of America, Washington, DC 20017.

Rehabilitation Gazette, International Journal and Information Service for the Disabled, 4502 Maryland Ave., St. Louis, MO 63108. (Also available on cassette or tape.)

The Indian Practitioner, Sassoon Building, 3rd Floor, 143, MG Road, Bombay-400 023.

Up Front, a newsletter for handicapped and disabled persons, 55 W. Park Ave., New Haven, CT 06511. 376 Bay 44th St., Brooklyn, NY 11214.

Books

Your local bookstores and libraries have many books on arthritis and other health-related subjects. Here are a few titles to get you started on a reading programme:

Barnard, Christian, M.D., *Christian Barnard's Program for Living with Arthritis*, Fireside/Simon & Schuster, New York, 1984.

Carr, Rachel, *Arthritis: Relief Beyond Drugs*, Harper & Row, New York, 1981.

Jetter, Judy and Nancy Kadlec, *The Arthritis Book of Water Exercise*, Holt, Rinehart and Winston, New York, 1985.

Krewer, Semyon, *The Arthritis Exercise Book*, Cornerstone Library/Simon & Schuster, New York, 1981.

Kushner, Irving M.D., *Understanding Arthritis*, Charles Scribner's Sons, New York, 1984.

Lunt, Suzanne, *A Handbook for the Disabled: Ideas and Inventions for Easier Living*, Charles Scribner's Sons, New York, 1982.

Mandell, Marshall, M.D., *Dr. Mandell's Lifetime Arthritis Relief System*, Berkley, New York, 1985.

Phillips, Robert, Ph.D., *Coping With Rheumatoid Arthritis*, Avery Publishing Group, Garden City Park, NY, 1988.

Scala, James, Ph.D., *The Arthritis Relief Diet*, new American Library, New York, 1987.

Schumacher, H. Ralph Jr., M.D., *Primer on the Rheumatic Diseases, Ninth Edition*, Atlanta, The Arthritis Foundation, GA, U.S.A., 1988.

Sobel, Dava and Arthur C. Klein, *Arthritis : What Works*, St. Martin's Press, New York, 1989.

Wade, Carlson, *How to Beat Arthritis with Immune Power Boosters*, Parker Publishing Company, West Nyack, NY, 1989.

Wallace, Jean, Ph.D., *Arthritis Relief*, PA, Rodale Press, Emmaus, 1989.

Engleman, Ephraim P., M.D., and Milton Silverman, PhD. *Arthritis Book: A Guide for Patients and Their Families,* Painter-Hopkins, Sausalito, CA, 1979.

Fries, James F., M.D., *Arthritis: A comprehensive Guide.* Addison-Wesley Publishing Co., Reading MA, 1979.

Reamy, Lois, *Travel Ability,* Macmillan Publishing Co., Inc., New York, 1978.

Robinson, Harold Speers, M.D., *You Asked about Rheumatoid Arthritis,* Douglas & McIntyre, Vancouver, BC, Canada, 1978.

Rosenberg, Alan M., M.D., *Living with Your Arthritis,* Arco Publishing, New York, 1979.

Ziebell, Beth, Ph.D., *As Normal as possible,* Arthritis Foundation, Southern Arizona Chapter, Tucson, AZ, 1976.

Combined Resources Will Be Effective

A combination of resources is available to help you understand your arthritis, cope with it every day, and possibly meet others who have similar concerns. Use these resources. They can help you help yourself to better health.

Glossary

Abduction : The movement of a limb away from the central axis of the body.

Acetabulum : The cup-shaped socket in the hipbone into which the head of the femur (the large bone between the knee and hip, also knows as the thighbone) fits.

Acromegaly : A hormonal disease resulting from excessive secretion of *human growth hormone,* which regulates growth. Excessive amounts of growth hormone can cause bones and soft tissues to thicken, resulting in osteoarthritis.

Adrenocorticotropic Hormone (ACTH): Produced by the pituitary gland, a small gland at the base of the brain, ACTH stimulates the release of cortisol and other natural steroid hormones from the adrenal glands. Some physicians use ACTH injections to treat arthritis, though the practice is not common.

Adduction : The movement of a limb toward the central axis of the body: the opposite of abduction (see definition).

Agglutination Test : A technique used to detect the presence of a variety of antibodies in the blood. For instance, the presence of rheumatoid factor (an antibody) in the blood is usually detected through an agglutination test. When the results of this test are positive an aggregation or clump, visible through a microscope (or often the naked eye), forms.

Alignment: The naturally correct positions of all parts of the body.

Allopurinol: The generic name for a drug that blocks the formation of uric acid in the body, used in the treatment of gout.

Anemia: A decreased level of red blood cells or haemoglobin in the bloodstream. An antibody reaction or other effects of arthritis can reduce the number of red blood cells in the body and lead to anemia.

Antibody: A protein responsible for immunity made by a type of white blood cell called a plasma cell. The antibody defends the body by fighting off foreign particles called *antigens* (see definition) and thus helps prevent infection. The second time the body encounters these foreign antigens it is better prepared and produces antibodies both faster and in greater numbers than on the first response.

Antigens: Foreign *invaders* in the body, such as bacteria, fought by one's antibodies when the body's immune system is working effectively.

Arthralgia: Pain in a joint in the absence of signs or symptoms of inflammation.

Arthritis: A disease characterized by the inflammation of one or more joints; there are more than 100 different types. The joints may become warmer than usual and show redness, swelling, pain and tenderness.

Arthrodesis: A process through which portions of an otherwise very unstable and deformed joint are surgically removed and the joint is fused and permanently locked into its most useful position.

Arthrogram: An X-ray technique for examining joints. A contrast medium (either air or a liquid, opaque to X-ray) is injected into the joint space, allowing its outline and contents to be traced accurately. The machine for taking out the arthrogram is called arthroscope.

Arthroplasty: A process of joint reconstruction that involves surgically rebuilding or modifying a joint or replacing it with an artificial joint.

Articular Cartilage: See Cartilage.

Autoimmune Disease: A disease in which a person's antibodies, which normally attack only "nonself" or foreign antigens, attack his or her own body. Some researchers say that systemic lupus erythematosus (SLE) may be one such disease.

Azathioprine: The generic name of an immunosuppressant drug that slows the progression of rheumatoid arthritis in some patients. Short-term side effects seem relatively uncommon, though it has not yet been determined what effects the drug may have in the long term.

Bacteria: Bacteria are tiny single-celled or noncellular organisms. They exist in great variety. Some need air to exist, while others do not; they may subsist through a great range of temperatures and require a variety of nutrients. While some are utterly harmless or even beneficial, others are extremely deadly. Bacteria may invade the joints and produce infectious arthritis.

Biofeedback: A technique through which an individual is constantly provided with information on the state of one or more of his or her body processes, using monitoring devices. This is done with the hope of altering these normally involuntary processes, possibly through conscious effort.

Blood Count: The determination of the number of red or white blood cells in a given volume of blood.

Bunion: A swelling on the first joint of the big toe that may be bony or due to bursitis.

Bursa: A small fluid-filled sac lined with a thin membrane that allows tendons to move smoothly over bones.

Bursitis: Inflammation of a bursa that most frequently affects the shoulder but may occur in other joints such as hips and elbows. Symptoms of bursitis are similar to those of arthritis, and correct diagnosis is important. Irritation from pressure or injury can cause inflammation of a bursa. Tenderness, pain, redness, and swelling may occur. Treatment may include drugs, injections of corticosteroids, rest, physical therapy, and, in some cases surgery.

Capsulectomy: Capsulectomy is the removal of the joint capsule, the fibrous membrane that covers a movable joint.

Cartilage: A thin tissue that covers opposing ends of bones within a joint and allows for relatively frictionless movement between the bones.

Cervical: Referring to the neck or that region of the body.

Chrysotherapy: The treatment of rheumatoid arthritis with injections of gold salts.

Colchicine: The generic name of a drug used to treat attacks of gout and to prevent gout from recurring. The drug is useful for few other types of arthritis and has many side effects. Because most patients who respond to colchicine have gout, the drug may help your doctor pinpoint the type of arthritis you have. After that you may be advised to switch to one of the other antiinflammatory drugs.

Collagen: A tough, fibrous protein occurring as a major component of connective tissues such as tendons, ligaments, cartilage and bone.

Collagen Diseases: Diseases characterized by alteration of connective tissues, such as inflammtion or degeneration. Rheumatoid arthritis and systemic lupus erythematosus (SLE) are two examples of collagen diseases.

Connective Tissue: These tissues, such as ligaments and tendons, support the body.

Cortisone: A steroid hormone produced by the adrenal gland and also produced synthetically. It can be used to reduce pain and swelling in arthritis. Its side effects can be very serious, especially when it is given daily over a period longer than two months.

Degenerative Arthritis: A chronic type of arthritis resulting from a degeneration of cartilage and bone; also called *osteoarthritis*. This is also referred to as *old age arthritis* and is the most common form of arthritis.

Drug Interaction: A process whereby one drug cancels or heightens the other's effects to a dangerous point when two drugs are incompatible with each other. Also, the combination of drugs may be poisonous.

Edema: A swelling of the tissues that takes place when too much fluid accumulates in various parts of the body.

Extension: The straightening of a joint.

Fascitis: Inflammation of the fibrous tissue known as *Fascia*, which is closely linked to muscle.

Femoral Head: The upper part of the femur thighbone.

Fenoprofen: The generic name for a nonsteroidal antiinflammatory drug (an NSAID).

Fibrinogen: A protein necessary to the clotting of blood.

Fibroblasts: Connective tissue cells commonly found in developing or repairing tissues, where they build the connective tissues.

Fibrocartilage: A dense, fibrous connective tissue in which small masses of cartilage exist between the fibres.

Fibrositis: A combination of unexplained complaints of pains, tender points, and stiffness throughout the body. The cause of fibrositis is most frequently not found; however, in many people, fibrositis is due to a lack of deep sleep.

Flexion Contracture: A condition in which the muscles and ligaments are shortened or tightened so that a joint cannot be straightened.

Gold Salts: Effective drugs for some patients with rheumatoid arthritis; have been shown to produce a remission of arthritis in some patients.

Gout: A form of arthritis caused by crystals of uric acid in the joints. These crystals are present only after prolonged elevation of uric acid in the serum.

Hamstrings: The tendons at the back of the knee.

Heberden's Nodes: Heberden's nodes are small bony growths on the end joints of the fingers. These nodes are usually a sign of osteoarthritis.

Haemoglobin: The protein in red blood cells that carries oxygen.

Haemophilia: A hereditary disease that occurs in males and is marked by impaired blood clotting and easy bleeding. If bleeding occurs in a joint, arthritis may develop and the joint may degenerate.

Hydroxychloroquine: An antimalarial drug that is useful in treating rheumatoid arthritis. Because of the remote possibility of eye damage, patients taking hydroxychloroquine should have an eye examination every six months.

Ibuprofen: The generic name of a nonsteroidal antiinflammatory drug (NSAID)used in various types of arthritis.

Indomethacin: The generic name of a nonsteroidal antiinflammatory drug (NSAID)used in the treatment of arthritis.

Infectious Arthritis: A form of arthritis caused by bacteria. Since antibiotics can kill bacteria, infectious arthritis is protentially curable.

Intervertebral Disc: Pieces of fibrocartilage that separate and cushion the vertebrae.

Iris: The coloured part of the eye. Like a camera's shutter, it controls the amount of light entering the eye. In juvenile rheumatoid arthritis the iris may be affected, possibly impairing vision or causing blindness.

Isometric Exercise: A type of exercise in which the contractions of the muscles are checked by opposing muscles and the muscles are stregthened without bending the joint.

Kyphosis: A term for humpback.

Ligament: A fibrous band of connective tissue that holds two bones together.

Lordosis: A forward curvature of the lower spine.

Lumbago: A general term for a lower backache.

Lumbar: Refers to the lower back.

Lymphocyte: A type of white blood cell involved in the body's immune response.

Muscle: Tissues that expand or contract. There are three types of muscle. *Striated,* or *skeletal* muscle are the most common type and enable movement of the bones and joints. *Smooth* muscle is involuntary muscle. Two examples are muscle that line the blood vessels and breathing passages. Cardiac muscle is found only in the heart and never rests.

Musculoskeletal: A term that applies to both the muscular and skeletal systems.

Myositis: Inflammation of a muscle, usually a strainted muscle, which causes weakness and sometimes pain and tenderness.

Naproxen: The generic name of a non-steroidal antiinflammatory drug used in arthritis. They are more expensive than aspirin. While the NSAIDs are not more effective than aspirin, they may have fewer side effects. *Nonsteroidal* is important here since it indicates that these drugs are not steroids.

Osteoarthritis: Another term for degenerative arthritis, a disease that is more likely to occur as one grows older and involves progressive deterioration of cartilage and bone in the joints.

Osteomyelitis: Bacterial infection of bone.

Osteoporosis: A term that refers to the thinning of bone. As the structure of the bone weakens, it becomes very brittle. Over long term use, steroids can lead to osteoporosis.

Osteotomy: The surgical procedure of cutting a bone to correct a deformity, thereby reducing pain and further deformity.

Oxyphenbutazone: The generic term for a nonsteroidal antiinflammatory drug used to treat arthritis.

Phenylbutazone: The generic name for a nonsteroidal antiinflammatory drug used to treat arthiritis.

Probenecid: The generic name for a drug used in the treatment of gout that lowers the level of uric acid in the blood by increasing its elimination by the kidneys. Aspirin prevents probenecid from working and therefore should not be used at the same time.

Prosthesis: An artificial body part. In arthritis, joint prostheses are sometimes used.

Psoriatic Arthritis: About one of 20 cases of psoriasis, a skin disease, is complicated by a form of arthritis. Treatment for psoriatic arthritis is similar to that for rheumatoid arthritis.

Purine: A product of nucleic acid metabolism that is the precursor of uric acid. Therefore, gout patients should limit foods containing purines, such as sweetbreads, liver, kidney, and brains (see Chapter 6).

Quadriceps: Large muscles along the front of the thighs.

Red Blood Cells: Cells that transport oxygen to the tissues and remove carbon dioxide.

Reiter's Syndorme: In 1916 Hans Reiter described the triad of arthritis, urethritis and conjunctivitis which came to be known by his name. Reiter's syndrome is now classified as a form of reactive arthritis. The joints most frequently affected are in succession, the knee ankle, hip and small joints of the hands and feet. These become swollen and painful. Involvement of the skin is common in the form of rupture with a thick horny crust. This is most marked on the soles of the feet.

Rheumatic Fever: A form of arthritis that very occasionally occurs after sore thorat. Rheumatic fever is characterized by high fever and inflammation of connective tissues, mainly in the heart and joints.

Rheumatism: A broad term used to describe inflammation, stiffness, and tenderness of the muscle or joints.

Rheumatoid Arthritis: A chronic disease of unknown cause, that generally occurs throughout the whole body. It causes pain and inflammation of the joints, limits their range of motion, and in some patients slowly destroys them. While there is no cure for rheumatoid arthritis, it can be treated and controlled.

Rheumatoid Factor: An antibody found in rheumatoid arthritics' blood that causes clumping of cells in the agglutination test for rheumatoid arthritis.

Rotation: The movement of a joint in a circular motion.

Sacroiliac Joint: A joint that connects the hipbones and the lower part of the spine.

Salicylates: A family of drugs used in arthritis for their powerful antiinflammatory effects and their ability to reduce pain. Aspirin is the most common of salicylates.

Scleroderma: A disease of the body's connective tissues. Usually, there is a thickening and hardening of the skin and sometimes inflammatory and other changes in internal organs, such as the esophagus, intestinal tract, heart, lungs, and kidneys.

Scoliosis: A sideways deviation in a normally vertically straight spine.

Spondylitis: Arthritis of the spine.

Staphylococcus: Bacteria that are very prevalent and are often associated with infectious arthritis.

Steroid Hormones: Hormones that include the sex hormones *androgen* and *estrogen* and the corticosteroids.

Streptococcus: Bacteria that cause severe infections and may be associated with infectious arthritis.

Synovectomy: Removal of the synovial membrane from an inflamed joint.

Synovial Fluid: A clear viscous liquid produced by the synovial membrane, which lubricates movable joints and contains nutrients for cartilage.

Synovial Membrane: A sheet of tissue found in joints, bursas, and tendon sheaths.

Systemic Lupus Erythematosus (SLE): A disease of inflammation of many parts of the body such as the joints, skin, kidneys, heart, brain and lungs.

Temporal Arthritis: It occurs in the elderly and most commonly affects the arteries of the scalp. The patient complains of severe headache, and blindness may result from thrombosis of the arteries to the eyes.

Tendon: A dense, fibrous connective tissue that attaches a bone and muscle together so that the bone moves when the muscle contracts.

Tenotomy: The cutting of a tendon.

Tolmetin Sodium: The generic name for a nonsteroidal antiinflammatory drug.

Tophi: Lumps of uric acid crystals that have been deposited in the joints of the hands and feet, the elbows, and the earlobes; a sign of gout.

Toxin: Any poisonous substance formed by plant or animal cells.

Traction: Drawing or pulling an extremity or joint to relieve pressure or realign the bones.

Transcutaneous Nerve Stimulation (TNS): A technique that stops messages such as pain along nerve pathways on their way to the brain by using an outside low-intensity current.

Trauma: Physical or psychological shock or an injury or wound.

Triceps: The large muscle along the back of the arm.

Ulnar Deviation: A deformation of the hand in the direction of the little finger.

Ultrasound Therapy: Therapy that uses high-frequency sound waves to produce heat in tissues under the skin in order to relieve pain.

Uric Acid: A product of purine metabolism; too much uric acid in the blood over a prolonged period of time (years) can lead to the development of gout.

Uricosuric Drugs: Drugs that increase the kidney's excretion of uric acid.

Vertebrae: Bones (33 of them) in the spinal column.

Virus: Tiny structures (not cells) made up of a core of nucleic acid surrounded by a protein sheath. They depend entirely on living cells for reproduction, as they have no metabolism of their own. In invading living cells, viruses can cause infection.

While Blood Cells: The blood cells concerned with defending the body against infection and disease; also known as leukocytes.

Index

174

High Blood Cholesterol:
Causes, Prevention & Treatment

Dr Krishan Gupta MD, MRCP, FACP   Rs 65.00
Prof. of Clinical Medicine, New York Medical College, USA

The book tells you how high blood cholesterol can be prevented and controlled. It recommends practical tips for choosing the right foods and suggests Dos and Don'ts of a low cholesterol lifestyle.

"If you have high cholesterol levels, get hold of this book."

–Times of India

Cancer:
Causes, Prevention & Treatment

Dr O.P. Jaggi, MD, Ph.D   Illus.   Rs 60.00

This straightforward and helpful book tells you how early detection and aggressive treatment *can* and *does* save life.

Asthma & Allergies:
Causes, Prevention & Treatment

Dr O.P. Jaggi, MD, Ph.D   Illus.   Rs 70.00

"A comprehensive and readily understandable book . . . a must for doctors, post-graduates and general practitioners. This book is useful also to patients of chronic asthma."

–The Hindu

Diabetes:
Causes, Prevention & Treatment

Ada P. Kahn, MPH   Rs 65.00

"In this book you will learn about the many aspects of diabetes and its treatment. The author presents up-to-date information clearly enough to help you better understand your disease."

– Dr Melvin M Chertrack, MD
Past President American Diabetes Association